T0146029

RAND

Testing CAHPS® Health Plan Performance Reports in the Florida Medicaid Program

*Donna O. Farley, Pamela Farley Short,
David E. Kanouse, Diane Schoeff,
Julie A. Brown, Mark Spranca, and
Ron D. Hays*

Prepared for the Agency for Healthcare Research and Quality

PREFACE

The Agency for Health Care Policy and Research (AHCPR), now the Agency for HealthCare Research and Quality, AHRQ), initiated the Consumer Assessment of Health Plans Study (CAHPS) project in 1995 to develop and test methods to provide consumers with comparative information on health plan performance. In partnership with the AHCPR, the CAHPS project has been carried out by a consortium of organizations, including RAND, Harvard Medical School and Research Triangle Institute. The consortium has developed and tested survey methods and reporting formats in field demonstrations in a variety of settings, including Medicaid programs, large employers, and health plan purchasing coalitions.

This report describes the findings from a demonstration that RAND conducted with the Florida Medicaid program to test applications of CAHPS consumer reports in the Medicaid sector. This demonstration was the first of RAND's CAHPS demonstrations. In collaboration with the Florida Agency for Health Care Administration (AHCA), we designed both paper and computer-based report formats, which were tested in field applications in Volusia County, Florida.

This research was supported through cooperative agreement No. 5U18HS09204-05 entitled "Consumer Assessments of Health Plans Study" from the Agency for Healthcare Research and Quality (AHRQ). Opinions are those of the authors and do not necessarily reflect the view of AHRQ or the affiliated institutions.

CONTENTS

TABLES

FIGURES

SUMMARY

This report describes the findings from a demonstration conducted by RAND with the Florida Medicaid program to test applications of Consumer Assessment of Health Plans Study (CAHPS®)[1] consumer reports in the Medicaid sector. In collaboration with the Florida Agency for Health Care Administration (AHCA), we designed both paper and computer-based report formats, which were tested in field applications in Volusia County, Florida. This demonstration was the first of RAND's CAHPS demonstrations. Results of this work have been applied in subsequent demonstrations with the New Jersey and Iowa Medicaid programs.

The Agency for Health Care Policy and Research, now the Agency for Healthcare Research and Quality (AHRQ), initiated the CAHPS project in 1995 to develop and test methods to provide consumers with comparative information on performance of health plans as reported by current health plan enrollees. The CAHPS project has been carried out by a consortium of organizations under a cooperative agreement with the AHRQ, including RAND, Harvard Medical School, the Research Triangle Institute, and Westat. The consortium has developed survey methods and reporting formats and has tested them in field demonstrations in a variety of settings, including Medicaid programs, large employers, and health plan purchasing coalitions. The demonstrations are aimed at improving the CAHPS surveys and reports and determining the usefulness of CAHPS products to consumers and purchasers.

The CAHPS reporting dimensions consist of global ratings by consumers (e.g. rating of the plan or primary care provider) and reports about how well a plan performed on specific functions (e.g. getting care when needed or provider treating the patient with respect). The CAHPS consortium developed *stars* and *bars* formats to display comparative health plan information on each performance dimension. The stars show how each plan performed on a CAHPS dimension compared to all the other health plans in a CAHPS survey. The bars display the plans' quantitative survey results for each CAHPS dimension (expressed as percentage of responses).

The Florida AHCA is responsible for a range of health-related government functions, including administration of the Florida Medicaid program that serves approximately 1.4 million clients. The Medicaid program has introduced mandatory managed care enrollment for many of its Medicaid recipients, under which new Medicaid recipients have a choice of a primary care case management option (called MediPass) or one of the Medicaid health maintenance organizations (HMOs). AHCA fielded a preliminary version of the CAHPS survey in late 1996 with samples of enrollees in Medicaid and private sector health plans.

In this report, we document the entire demonstration that RAND performed in collaboration with the Florida AHCA to field test report formats to present CAHPS information for Medicaid recipients. Two report formats were tested in one Florida county: a paper report mailed with the standard Medicaid enrollment materials, and a computer-based report installed in the reception area of a local Economic Services office for welfare recipients. In Section 2, we describe the design of each of these report formats, and in Section 3 we describe the methods we used to evaluate the field tests of the reports. The next two sections present the results of the

---

[1] Registered trademark of the Agency for Healthcare Research and Quality for the Consumer Assessment of Health Plans Study.

fields tests for the paper report (Section 4) and the computer-based report, called the Decision Helper (Section 5). Finally, we summarize in Section 6 the key issues and implications of the Florida field test findings for future CAHPS reporting applications.

HIGHLIGHTS OF FINDINGS

The Florida Medicaid demonstration yielded a broad range of valuable information that has helped guide subsequent CAHPS demonstration and reports applications across the country. We summarize here selected findings that we believe stand out as some of the key lessons from this early demonstration. Although some lessons emerged from field testing the paper report and others from testing the Decision Helper, these findings cut across both reporting media:

- Consumers expressed *some distrust of the plan performance reports*. Some felt that group averages did not apply to them, some were concerned that performance measures were not developed independently but were influenced by health plans, and others did not fully understand how information from a survey sample can be valid for a larger population.

- *Ease of access to and use of information* is critical to ensure that performance reports are useful and consumers will use them. For both paper reports and the Decision Helper, this means short, clear sentences in the instructions, explanations on how to use the measures, and tables of measures that can be read easily and quickly. In addition, the Decision Helper computer screens need to be easy to understand, the navigational path through the screens must be easy to follow, and navigational instructions must conform to locations on the screen where people look first.

- For maximum effect, the *timing of access to plan performance information* should coincide with the point in time when consumers are making their health plan decisions (neither too early nor too late).

- Two key findings were unique to the computer-based system. First, *computer literacy was not a barrier* to using the Decision Helper for Florida Medicaid recipients because many already had experience with computers, ATMs, and video games. Second, it is important to establish a *physical environment that provides privacy* during use of the Decision Helper, or people will be discouraged from using it.

- For all performance report applications, successful implementation will be determined by paying *careful attention to details* — not only of the performance measures, but also of the layout and design of the report, the method for disseminating the reports to consumers, and the timing and reliability of the dissemination actions.

OVERVIEW OF THE DEMONSTRATION

The information reported in the Medicaid paper report and Decision Helper tested in the demonstration was drawn from the 1996 AHCA survey results for the Medicaid enrollee sample. Our goal was to achieve report formats that were easy to use for Florida Medicaid recipients and that provided useful information for their health plan choices. All work was performed during the latter half of 1997, with design of the paper report starting in May 1997 and design of the Decision Helper starting in June 1997. Field applications for both reports took place late in the year, as did RAND's evaluation activities.

We decided to limit the field test of the reports to one county within the state. The selection of a field test location for the Decision Helper drove the choice of county for testing the paper report. We decided to place the Decision Helper in an Economic Services Office because they are the only locations where large percentages of Medicaid recipients use the system. Using selection criteria and findings from visits to the sites, we chose the Daytona Beach office as the field test location for the Decision Helper. Therefore, paper reports were mailed to new recipients residing in Volusia County (in which Daytona Beach is located).

RAND developed the plan ratings report as a separate document to be added to the mailing materials to new Medicaid recipients. AHCA already provided Medicaid recipients with a report entitled *The Choice Is Yours* that contained information on the managed care program. The plan rating booklet, which we entitled *Here Are Your Choices—Medicaid Health Plans in Volusia County*, contained background information about the survey that generated the ratings information, descriptions of MediPass and Medicaid HMOs, instructions on how to use the report, and survey results for each plan offered in Volusia County. Using AHCA survey data, we established two overall rating measures and eight composite groupings. The report also provided some guidance on making a plan choice and questions to ask when choosing a health plan.

The *Here Are Your Choices* booklet used a full 8.5" by 11" page layout to display information, and it was folded once to make it the same 8.5" by 5.5" size as *The Choice Is Yours* document. This design allowed the booklet to fit into the 6" x 9" envelope used for mailing Medicaid enrollment materials. To minimize costs for printing materials, the booklet was prepared in black and white, duplicated on a copy machine, given a green cover, and stapled together in the top right corner. The booklets were distributed in mailings to new Medicaid recipients in Volusia County during November and December 1997.

The adaptation of the Decision Helper for a Medicaid population was performed during the summer 1997. Field testing of the Medicaid Decision Helper in the Daytona Beach Economic Services Office began in early October. Our starting template was the CAHPS Decision Helper model developed for the privately insured population. Understanding the need to make the system easy to use for Medicaid beneficiaries, we demonstrated the CAHPS Decision Helper with the staff of AHCA, the Medicaid program, and Economic Services program to seek their feedback. Participants believed that the system needed to be simplified substantially for the Medicaid population, and they provided detailed comments on individual screen displays. Working with this feedback, the RAND team designed the Florida Medicaid Decision Helper.

EVALUATION METHODS

In our evaluations of the Florida Medicaid paper report and the Decision Helper, we wanted to obtain information from the major stakeholders involved in use of these reports. AHCA and the Medicaid program were obvious stakeholders, as sponsors of the survey and consumer reports. Others included Medicaid recipients who would use these reports and Medicaid health plans whose performances were being compared. In addition, the state and local Economic Services Offices were important stakeholders for field placements of the Decision Helper in local Economic Services Offices.

We undertook three major evaluation tasks to obtain information from each major stakeholder. First, we evaluated the use of the Decision Helper in the Daytona Beach office, including observations of use of the system, exit interviews of users, and analysis of daily use logs generated by the Decision Helper software. Second, we conducted focus groups with Medicaid recipients to obtain consumer feedback on the paper report. Third, after completion of the field tests of the paper report and Decision Helper, two RAND staff conducted a 2-day site visit to Florida and performed individual and group interviews with representatives of AHCA, the Medicaid program, Economic Services Offices, the MediPass program, and the two HMOs serving Volusia County.

EVALUATION RESULTS

The Florida Medicaid demonstration revealed several issues involved in effective communication with Medicaid consumers that were common to both paper report and Decision Helper media. Four general dimensions of a consumer information strategy were identified during the demonstration:

- The types, amounts, and display of the plan performance information itself;
- The design of the report medium, including the paper report document and the software and hardware of the Decision Helper;
- The physical environment in which the information is provided to potential users; and
- The timing of information availability relative to when plan choices are being made.

In this demonstration, we examined the strengths and weaknesses of the paper and computer-based reports on each dimension of this framework. We found clear evidence that failures in any dimension can impede the communication process if the failures lead to consumers' not noticing the reports or discourage them from spending time with the information.

Paper Reports

The issue of trust in the survey information was prevalent in the focus group feedback about the paper report. Participants expressed concerns that the survey sample did not represent them as individuals, as well as concerns about the objectivity of the survey itself. Some participants who challenged the representativeness of the sample appeared to not fully understand the concept of random samples. Others challenged the sample because it was a mix of people who, on average, might have health plan or service needs that differed from an individual's specific needs. Some questions regarding the objectivity of the survey appeared to be motivated by suspicions that health plans may have influenced the survey results. The location of the survey information at the back of the *Here Are Your Choices* booklet appeared to have contributed to the trust issues, which might be alleviated by placing the survey information at the front of the booklet.

Other important feedback was participants' requests that the report contain information on the plan features and covered benefits, as well as the comparative performance information. Such a comprehensive presentation can help strengthen the plan choice process by giving beneficiaries easy access to the full set of information they should be considering.

The options for report layout were constrained by the Medicaid program's existing production and mailing requirements, resulting in a visually uninteresting document that was somewhat difficult to use. A more challenging issue is whether to produce one state-wide report or separate reports for individual counties or cluster of counties served by the same health plans.

Although the separate county reports would be more useful to beneficiaries, they would entail greater production, mailing, and administrative costs for the Medicaid program.

Decision Helper

The field test documented low use rates for the Decision Helper, with similar results obtained from our computer logs and the two-day observation period. From the observation period, we estimated that 8.4 percent of those entering the Economic Services Office approached the computer and only half of them used it for more than one minute. We had anticipated that only a fraction of potential users would find this medium attractive. However, use rates were lower than expected. Computer literacy did not appear to be a constraint for use of the Decision Helper, as reflected in reports by exit interview respondents of high use rates of computer-based systems. Close to 88 percent of respondents had used a computer, 74 percent had used an ATM, and 96 percent had played video games. We identified a number of factors that appeared to discourage use:

- Exit interview results showed that people who approached the Decision Helper after they had completed their case worker interviews were more likely to use it, compared with those who were still waiting for their appointments. The lower use before the case worker appointments may be because individuals thought they might be interrupted at the Decision Helper when called for their appointments. It also suggests that many Economic Service Office users may not yet be thinking about Medicaid and therefore may not be receptive to health plan information until reminded of it by their case workers.

- A few individuals reported in the exit interviews that they were embarrassed to use the Decision Helper. These responses suggest a privacy issue where some people may have been discouraged from using it if others in the waiting area could see what they were doing. Several individuals reported they did not want to be embarrassed by being observed making a mistake with the computer.

- Feedback generally reinforced the principle that "simpler is better" for both the contents of the information provided and navigational aspects of the system. Users responded positively to both the touch screen feature and the ability to print out pages to take home.

- Exit interview feedback highlighted the need to provide clear and simple instructions on how to use the system, ensure system speed so users can move quickly through the screens, and show a dialogue box confirming that a print request was being executed.

Other aspects of the Decision Helper product itself that we found needed careful management were the robustness of the system software and hardware and the daily maintenance requirements for the local office staff. Equipment security issues with respect to damage and theft were both more important and more complex than we had believed at the start of the field test. The demonstration also substantiated the need to have external technical expertise available to troubleshoot problems. However, because the Decision Helper was in daily operation for only 2 weeks before the on-site evaluation began, this placement did not fully test the viability of the system under long-term operating conditions.

DISCUSSION

Both the focus groups on the paper report and the exit interviews from the Decision Helper field test revealed that Florida Medicaid beneficiaries were interested in the comparative health plan information. Those interviewed tended to report they found the information to be useful and easy to interpret, although some were confused about interpretation of the stars. At the same time, participants expressed a diversity of opinions regarding the report contents, format, and timing of presentation.

This feedback from beneficiaries highlights the importance of continuing to build an foundation that defines the basic elements required to communicate plan performance information effectively, while allowing flexibility to tailor specific report design and dissemination to the preferences of each sponsor and the populations it serves. We understand there is no one "correct answer" for report design, yet empirical knowledge has not yet identified clearly which are the essential and discretionary elements for presentation.

The Florida demonstration also showed that multiple design and implementation factors can affect the success or failure of efforts to report CAHPS survey findings to consumers. This finding applies equally to both the paper report and Decision Helper, although successful field placement of the Medicaid Decision Helper involves the management of multiple, complex factors. Thus, evaluations should not be quick to generalize from the success or failure of any particular implementation of CAHPS (or consumer report cards more generally) because a slightly different implementation might have very different results. Furthermore, each CAHPS sponsor needs to exercise considerable care to make sure that their implementation is fine-tuned to the specifics of their particular situation.

The collective findings of the Florida Medicaid demonstration offer persuasive support for the premise that CAHPS and other plan performance information can provide value for Medicaid beneficiaries. Participants generally interpreted the stars effectively to make plan comparisons, and they tended to approach the task with a healthy skepticism that yielded realistic interpretations of the information before them. What effects this information may have on their actual health plan choices, however, remain to be tested before any conclusions can be drawn regarding the effects of CAHPS. Given the large size of the Medicaid populations across the states, Medicaid CAHPS could contribute substantially to helping large numbers of beneficiaries make more informed plan choices — if they choose to use the information.

ACKNOWLEDGEMENTS

It is a pleasure to acknowledge the contributions of the many people with whom we have worked on the Florida Medicaid demonstration for the CAHPS project, without whose participation we could not have gathered the valuable information this demonstration yielded. We thank the staff of the Florida Agency for Health Care Administration and Department of Families and Children for their active participation in the adaptation of CAHPS templates to the Florida Medicaid paper reports and Decision Helper, as well as their support throughout our field test activities. Particular thanks go to Russell Mardon and Kim Shafer, who were our AHCA points of contact for this work, both of whom were actively engaged throughout the demonstration and offered us valuable substantive and procedural guidance.

The field test of the Decision Helper would not have been a reality without the committed support by the leadership of the Daytona Beach Economic Services Office. Our appreciation goes to David Putnam and Lynne Sedmina, who provided the local leadership for the field test and ensured we had the support needed to install the computer system in the office waiting area, maintain daily operation, and perform our evaluation activities.

The "front line" work in adapting the template Decision Helper to the Florida Medicaid version was undertaken as a collaboration between Digital Evolution and two of our RAND colleagues, Terry West and Susan Phillips. We thank them for the commitment they made to delivering a solid computer-based product under stringent timelines, which was the basis for the Daytona Beach field test. Our appreciation also is offered to Matt Lewis for his fine field contributions for the installation of the Decision Helper in Daytona Beach, training for local staff, and ongoing support of the field application.

We also wish to acknowledge the contributions of the many individuals who reviewed earlier drafts of this report on the RAND Florida Medicaid demonstration. We thank Christine Crofton, one of our AHRQ project officers, and Lisa Meredith, our RAND colleague, for their thoughtful reviews of both substance and presentation of the demonstration findings. Their suggestions have made this a better document. We appreciate the on-going support and guidance of our AHRQ project officers, Christine Crofton and Charles Darby, throughout the CAHPS project, of which this demonstration was one component.

Section 1

THE FLORIDA MEDICAID CAHPS DEMONSTRATION

In October 1995, the Agency for Health Care Policy and Research (now the Agency for Healthcare Research and Quality, AHRQ) initiated the Consumer Assessment of Health Plans Study (CAHPS®) to develop and test methods to provide consumers with comparative information on performance of health plans as reported by current health plan enrollees. The CAHPS® project has been performed by a consortium of organizations under a cooperative agreement with the AHRQ, including RAND, Harvard Medical School, the Research Triangle Institute, and Westat. The consortium has developed survey methods and reporting formats and has tested them in field applications through demonstrations in both the public and private health insurance sectors.

This report describes the findings from a demonstration conducted by RAND with the Florida Medicaid program to test applications of CAHPS consumer reports in the Medicaid sector. In collaboration with the Florida State Agency for Health Care Administration (AHCA), we designed both paper and computer-based report formats, which were tested in field applications in Volusia County, Florida. This was the first of RAND's CAHPS demonstrations. Results of this work have been applied in subsequent demonstrations with the New Jersey and Iowa Medicaid programs. In this Section, we first provide an overview of the CAHPS project, followed by a description of RAND's demonstration with the Florida Medicaid program. Then we discuss our process and logic for selecting Volusia County for the demonstration site. Finally, we provide a "roadmap" for material covered in the remaining chapters of the report.

THE CONSUMER ASSESSMENT OF HEALTH PLANS STUDY

The overall goal of CAHPS is to provide an integrated set of tested and standardized survey questionnaires and accompanying report formats that can be used to collect and report information from enrollees about their health plan experiences. These materials have been designed for use with all types of health insurance enrollees (Medicaid and Medicare beneficiaries as well as the privately insured) and across the full range of health care delivery systems, from fee-for-service to managed care plans. The information from CAHPS questionnaires and reports can help consumers and group purchasers compare health plans to make more informed plan choices. The CAHPS templates for report formats have been developed using extensive cognitive interview and focus group methods, as well as field testing in demonstration settings. Reporting needs guided the design of items and composite measures included in the CAHPS surveys, with one of the goals being to minimize cognitive burden (McGee, et al., 1999).

The AHRQ made an early commitment to field demonstrations to test CAHPS products in a variety of settings, including Medicaid programs, large employers, and health plan purchasing coalitions. In the demonstration sites, CAHPS survey instruments and reporting formats have been used to collect and report information to the public. Members of the CAHPS teams have provided technical assistance and performed process and outcome evaluations of the CAHPS products. These field tests were aimed at improving the CAHPS surveys and reports and determining the usefulness of CAHPS products to consumers and purchasers in selecting health care plans and services (Crofton, Lubalin, & Darby, 1999).

The CAHPS dimensions consist of global ratings by consumers (e.g. rating of the plan, rating of personal doctor or nurse) as well as reports about how well a plan performed in specific areas (e.g. getting care when needed or provider treating the patient with respect). The CAHPS version 1.0 contained four global ratings (scale of 0 to 10) and nine report composites. These dimensions were streamlined in CAHPS version 2.0 to two global ratings and five report composites. The CAHPS consortium developed two formats for displaying comparative health plan information on each of these performance dimensions:

- *Stars* - show how each plan performed on a CAHPS dimension compared to all the other health plans for which a sponsor surveyed enrollees. Based on tests of statistical significance (and also of practical significance if desired by the sponsor), a health plan is given one star if it has a lower average score on a dimension than the average for all other plans, and it is given three stars if it has a higher average score. Otherwise the plan gets two stars for that dimension.

- *Bar chart* - display the quantitative survey results (expressed as percentage of responses) for all the plans for each CAHPS dimension.

The computer-based report format developed in CAHPS, called the Decision Helper, provides consumer rating and report information in an automated system with which users can interact as they consider their health plan options. Our field test of the Decision Helper as part of the Florida Medicaid demonstration was the first of the Medicaid field applications of the computer-based system. It was designed to examine the feasibility of such a system and to test the system design and field conditions necessary for successful implementation in a Medicaid environment.

CONCEPTUAL FRAMEWORK

Any test of the effects of consumer rating information on people's health plan choices needs to be performed within the framework of what we already know about the factors people consider in choosing plans. The plan characteristics that are important to consumers have been studied extensively over the years. Studies typically have collected data on self-reported preferences, using such methods as survey or focus groups, or have estimated analytic models of the effects of various factors on actual plan enrollment choices. Several key factors found consistently to be important to consumers are the health benefits offered, costs to the consumer, maintaining established providers, and freedom of provider choice (Mechanic, et al., 1990; Marquis and Rogowski, 1991; Davis, et al., 1995; Scanlon, et al., 1997, Sainfort and Booske, 1996; Gibbs, et al., 1996; Tumlinson, et al., 1997). Some inconsistency also has been found, however, in that the factors that individuals report as being important to them differ from those they actually use to choose health plans (Mechanic, et al., 1989).

Although consumers have been found to use plan performance information in making plan choices, evidence has been mixed with respect to how they use it and its relative importance to them (Hibbard, et al.; 1996; Scanlon et al., 1997). Research findings suggest that consumers value information on quality factors such as HEDIS effectiveness of care indicators, physician board certification, waiting time for appointments, ease of getting specialty care, and disenrollment due to dissatisfaction. However, when making health plan choices, consumers place less priority on some of these quality factors than on benefits, provider choice or costs

(Sainfort and Booske, 1996; Castles, et al., 1997; Knutson, et al., 1997; Robinson and Brodie, 1997; Tumlinson et al., 1997; Chernew and Scanlon, 1998). In addition, consumer focus group participants have reported they do not understand consumer survey methods or how to interpret survey results, and some do not accept results as relevant to themselves. Similar concerns were identified for quality of care indicators (Gibbs, et al., 1996). Consumers often do not understand plan performance measures, and poorly understood measures are viewed as not being useful. Understanding tends to increase as consumers are exposed to the information and learn how to interpret it (Sainfort and Booske, 1996; Hibbard and Jewett, 1997). Thus, one strategy for reporting this information would be to design the reporting medium and process to help educate consumers on how to use the measures provided (Hibbard, et al.; 1997).

A Conceptual Model

The decision processes involved in making health plan choices involve interactions among a decision maker's own cognitive processes, the nature of the decision task, and the environmental or social context within which choices are being made. As a result, when introducing new information to the process, it may be difficult to discern the nature or direction of causality for changes in the decision process and resulting choices.

To guide our analysis for the CAHPS demonstrations, including field tests of report applications and assessments of the impacts of CAHPS information on plan choice, we use a conceptual model that defines the steps in this process and hypothesizes relationships among them. This model draws upon two theoretical frameworks for decision making: the *theory of adaptive decision making* and the *theory of utility and choice*. Extensive research efforts, including the literature discussed above, have generated empirical information on various aspects of these and other, similar models.

The *theory of adaptive decision making* defines a framework for how an individual chooses an approach for making a decision among alternatives—the first step in the decision process. According to this theory, individuals use different decision strategies under various circumstances, making tradeoffs between cognitive effort (cost of search) and the anticipated outcomes (benefits and risks) from that effort (Payne et al., 1993). Thus, individuals vary in the extent to which they seek information and types of information they consider.

The second step in the decision process is the act of choosing among alternatives, using the information collected. The *theory of utility and choice* addresses this step, stating that individuals make choices to achieve desired goals. Goal achievement is measured as maximizing utility by balancing preferences for multiple factors. When selecting a health plan, for example, an individual seeks an optimal combination of covered benefits, cost, quality, and risk protection based on his/her own preferences. For uncertain outcomes, expected utility is estimated by multiplying the utility of each outcome by the probability of the outcome occurring (Baron, 1988). This normative theory has been criticized for its underlying assumptions that choices are rational and fully informed. Indeed, research has shown that cognitive limitations, as well as risk aversion behavior, can lead to choices that differ from the "rational" choice among options.

Medicaid Managed Care

Managed care has become a central feature of Medicaid health coverage over the past decade, with state governments seeking ways to control costs while ensuring access to appropriate care for beneficiaries. Many state Medicaid programs now require beneficiaries who meet Aid to Families with Dependent Children (AFDC) criteria to enroll in a managed care plan, and growing numbers of states are extending these requirements to Supplemental Security Income (SSI) beneficiaries. Currently, all but 2 Medicaid programs have some form of mandatory or voluntary managed care program. As of June 1998, 585 health plans participated in Medicaid programs, serving more than 16 million beneficiaries or 54 percent of the nation's Medicaid population (HCFA, 1999). Medicaid beneficiaries are asked to choose a health plan from among some combination of traditional health maintenance organizations (HMO) and primary care case management models. In states with mandatory managed care, beneficiaries who do not make a voluntary choice are assigned a health plan by the Medicaid office (called auto-assignment).

The information needs and preferences of Medicaid populations in making health plan choices often are viewed as different from those of privately insured populations. Yet there is little empirical evidence regarding the existence or magnitudes of such differences. In recent laboratory experiments that simulated the plan choice process, both privately insured individuals and Medicaid beneficiaries who had CAHPS information were more likely to choose health plans that performed higher on the CAHPS results (Spranca, et al., 2000; Kanouse et al., in preparation). Although these results show that CAHPS® can affect Medicaid plan choices under controlled conditions, where beneficiaries are asked to consider this information, little is known about the extent to which similar effects would be observed when they receive plan performance information in the context of their normal daily lives, nor about how the communication medium may affect their use of the information.

Research Questions

Working from this conceptual framework, we wanted to test the field application of reports in the Florida Medicaid program to gain information on which factors may influence the extent to which these consumers integrate this new information into their choices of Medicaid health plans. Key research questions that we examined were:

- What are the requirements for successful implementation of plan performance reports in a Medicaid program, and how might they be managed?

- How readily can the CAHPS template for a report format be adapted for use with Medicaid populations?

- How receptive will Medicaid consumers be to reports containing plan performance information, and what factors are most likely to affect their receptivity?

- What features of a paper report are most (or least) important to Medicaid consumers?

- Do Medicaid recipients have the computer skills to use a computer-based system designed for assisting health plan choices, including provision of plan performance information?

- What are the optimal circumstances (location, timing, physical setup) for making a computerized system available to Medicaid recipients?

OVERVIEW OF THE DEMONSTRATION

The Florida State AHCA is responsible for a range of health-related functions within the Florida state government, including administration of the Medicaid program. The Florida

Medicaid program, which serves approximately 1.4 million clients across the state, has introduced mandatory managed care enrollment for many of its Medicaid recipients. As individuals enter Medicaid, they have a choice of a primary care case management option, called MediPass, or one of the health maintenance organizations (HMOs) that have contracted with Medicaid. Although Florida did not have an existing enrollment counseling program at the time of our demonstration, recently enacted State legislation required the establishment of such a program. Thus, the AHCA staff saw this demonstration as a potentially useful source of information to help guide their future program development efforts.

Our Florida Medicaid demonstration was designed to take advantage of the fact that AHCA fielded an early version of the CAHPS survey in late 1996, which included a sample of Medicaid recipients enrolled in 19 Medicaid health plans. With the availability of Florida Medicaid survey data early in the CAHPS demonstration activities, we were able to get an early start on adapting the paper report template and Decision Helper prototype for use with Medicaid populations.

For successful communications of CAHPS comparative health plan rating information, design of reports and dissemination methods need to accommodate a number of factors, including the number of health plan choices available, the integrity and usability of the report itself, the timing of information provision, and environmental conditions that may influence how much attention is paid to the information by potential users. We considered these factors in designing the paper and computer-based reports as well as in our selection of test site and report dissemination methods. In addition, we understood that health plans that were the subjects of the report would expect to be treated fairly in the presentation of their survey results. Therefore, we designed the Decision Helper pages that displayed performance information to be sure that all plans could be considered equally by users.

The RAND team worked in collaboration with AHCA to test the paper and computer-based report formats for a Medicaid population. Our goal was to achieve report formats that were easy to use for Florida Medicaid recipients and that provided them useful information for their health plan choices. RAND performed all the work involved in designing the paper report and computer-based Decision Helper for the Medicaid population. AHCA and the other Florida state agencies provided input to developing initial design specifications, and they reviewed preliminary designs and gave us feedback on revisions to better address issues they identified.

The schedule of tasks undertaken in the demonstration is presented in Table 1. All work was performed during the latter half of 1997, with design of the paper report starting in May 1997 and design of the Decision Helper starting in June 1997. Field applications for both reports took place late in the year, as did RAND's evaluation activities.

CHOICE OF THE DEMONSTRATION SITE

We decided to limit the field test of the reports to one county within the state. This strategy allowed us to focus on report design issues while minimizing the financial burden of the demonstration for AHCA. The selection of a location for field testing the Decision Helper drove the choice of county for testing the paper report because the paper report could be mailed easily to residents of any county whereas the requirements for a Decision Helper location were much more stringent.

Table 1
Florida Demonstration Schedule for the Paper Report and Decision Helper

Development Step	Month in 1997							
	May	June	July	Aug	Sept	Oct	Nov	Dec
Paper Report:								
Define composite groupings	▬							
Calculate composites		▬						
Basic report specifications		▬	▬					
First draft report prepared			▬	▬				
Review by AHCA				▬				
Revisions made by RAND					▬			
Final AHCA review					▬			
Camera ready report copy						▬		
Mail reports							▬	▬
Decision Helper:								
Florida review of prototype		▬						
Develop draft scripts			▬	▬				
Review by AHCA, ECS?					▬			
Prepare draft system				▬	▬			
Review by AHCA, ECS?						▬		
Final programming, taping						▬		
Field test in Daytona Beach						▬	▬	

The Florida Medicaid program does not have local offices to serve recipients because it communicates with Medicaid recipients solely via the U.S. mail and telephone. The only physical locations where large percentages of Medicaid recipients use the system are the local Economic Services Offices that administer the state welfare program. The Economic Services Offices are operated by a separate state agency, the Department of Children and Families (DCF). We decided that an Economic Services Office was the best available setting to test the Decision Helper. However, these offices are not ideal locations because (1) Medicaid-eligible persons using these offices are focusing on their welfare benefits and may not yet be ready to think about choosing a Medicaid health plan, and (2) some of the persons using the office for welfare benefits may not be candidates for Medicaid.

Because we were in the early phase of testing options for report format and contents, we wanted to focus our evaluation on the merits of the report itself and the modes of dissemination, controlling for variations in other factors. Therefore, we established the following criteria to select our Decision Helper field test site in Florida:

- offer Medicaid recipients a choice of 4 to 5 health plans;

- have a relatively small percentage of non-English-speaking population;

- be served by health plans that do not actively oppose reporting survey data to consumers;

- have substantial activity of AFDC and Medicaid enrollees in the local Economic Services Office that will generate a large enough sample within a week of field work to test our approach effectively, but not so much traffic as to impede access to the Decision Helper.

Using these selection criteria, AHCA identified two candidate locations for the Decision Helper: Daytona Beach in Volusia County, and Ocala in Marion County. Medicaid recipients in Daytona Beach had 3 plan choices, and those in Ocala had 4 choices. In July 1997, two members of RAND's team visited the Daytona Beach and Ocala Economic Services Offices to get acquainted with the personnel involved and observe office layouts and administrative procedures. In both offices, staff expressed moderate, but tentative, support for being a test site, yet expressed some concerns that it would add to their already heavy workloads. However, the management leadership of the Daytona Beach office viewed the concept of the Decision Helper enthusiastically and was quite interested in participating in the field test. Both offices met the criteria for sufficient traffic flow to gather data during a week of observation and exit interviews, and for small percentages of non-English speaking populations. Both offices also were converting to "one-stop shop" service centers for people eligible for a range of state benefits, in response to national welfare reform and other state initiatives. The availability of information on choices of Medicaid health plans fit nicely into this new model. Finally, both offices were receptive to the idea of AHCA installing a telephone by the computer for users to call the Medicaid office "800" number for questions or information (although AHCA subsequently decided that telephone placement was not feasible for the field test).

The Daytona Beach office was chosen as the field test location based primarily on the enthusiastic support expressed by its management leadership. The Daytona office staff were willing to allow the research team to test computerized sound and printing features for the Decision Helper. With such support, we expected to be able to test the full scope of the computer system design under favorable administrative conditions, with local office personnel working collaboratively with the RAND team during the field test period. Where problems are experienced under such favorable test conditions, we can conclude they would be yet more difficult in more typical situations.

ORGANIZATION OF THIS REPORT

In the remainder of this report, we document the entire demonstration that RAND performed in collaboration with the Florida AHCA to field test report formats for presenting CAHPS information for Medicaid recipients. In Section 2, we describe the design of each of these report formats, and in Section 3 we describe the methods we used to evaluate the field tests of the reports. The next two sections present the results of the fields tests for the paper report (Section 4) and the computer-based report, called the Decision Helper (Section 5). Finally, we summarize in Section 6 the key issues and implications of the Florida field test findings for future CAHPS reporting applications. Support documentation for the reports and our evaluation methods are presented in Appendices A through G.

Section 2

REPORT DESIGNS AND FIELD APPLICATIONS

We describe in this Section the steps taken by RAND and AHCA for the preparation and production of the paper report, design of the Decision Helper, and installation of the Decision Helper in the Daytona Beach Economic Services Office. Through our collaborative approach, we were able to generate products that were useful for the Florida Medicaid program and that also yielded valuable field test information for RAND to help strengthen the CAHPS products.

It was not possible to use the CAHPS version 1.0 ratings and report dimensions because the questionnaire used by AHCA for the Florida managed care survey was a preliminary version of the CAHPS questionnaire with many items that differed from those in the CAHPS 1.0 survey. Therefore, the first step the RAND team took was to derive domains based on the questions in the Florida survey, while striving to retain as much similarity to the CAHPS dimensions as possible. Using survey data provided by AHCA, we established two global rating measures and eight groupings of report items. The ratings and composite groupings and the survey items included in the composites are listed in Appendix A. Staff from AHCA and the Medicaid program reviewed these measures before they were finalized. Plan performance on these measures was presented in both the Florida Medicaid paper report and Decision Helper.

We describe first the methods used in preparing the paper report with the Florida AHCA survey results. Then we describe the design of the Decision Helper and its installation in the Daytona Beach Economic Services office in October 1997. These activities included interactions with several state-level agencies as well as with staff in the Daytona Beach office.

PREPARATION OF THE PAPER REPORT

The existing managed care brochure provided to new Medicaid recipients, entitled *The Choice Is Yours,* contained information on the mandatory managed care program, how to choose or change health plans, and what plans are available in each area of the state. This report used a question-and-answer format to present the information. It was a bi-lingual document, with one-half written in English and the other half in Spanish (flipped upside down). We were told by AHCA that the plan ratings and report information would have to be a separate document, rather than replacing the existing report with one that contained the existing information plus the plan performance information.

Before preparing the plan performance report, we reviewed the contents and format of *The Choice Is Yours* to be sure that the plan performance report complemented it and was accurate in presenting information on the Florida Medicaid program. In addition, the design of the actual performance report was influenced by two major factors: the need to fit it into the 6" x 9" envelope used for mailing Medicaid enrollment materials and a limited budget available for printing materials.

We gave the plan performance booklet the title *Here Are Your Choices-Medicaid Health Plans in Volusia County.* The booklet contained background information about the survey that produced the ratings information, descriptions of MediPass and Medicaid HMOs, instructions on how to use the report, and the reports and ratings for each plan offered in Volusia County. It also provided some guidance on how to make a plan choice and what questions to ask to help inform the choice. A copy of the document is presented in Appendix B. The contents were written to be no higher than a 7th to 8th grade reading level, and the page layout provided adequate "white space" to allow for easy reading.

The booklet contents were displayed in a full 8.5" by 11" page layout. The booklet was prepared in black and white, duplicated on a copy machine, and folded once to make it the same 8.5" by 5.5" size as *The Choice Is Yours* document. The booklet was given a green cover and was stapled together in the top right corner, so the staple was in the top left corner when the booklet was opened up for use.

The plan rating and report information was presented in the booklet using the CAHPS stars (described in Section 1). We used two formats to present the stars for the health plans offered in Volusia County. The first was a table that compared the three plans on the global ratings of the health plan itself and of the regular doctor or nurse. The second format was a series of pages, one for each health plan, that presented the plan's stars for the two global rating items as well as for the eight dimensions of health service delivery. The decision to present each plan's ratings on a separate page was intended to make the information more accessible for new Medicaid recipients. We believed this approach was useful in this situation, where only three plan options are available, but it could be more burdensome where many more choices were available. We tested display issues in the focus groups during our evaluation.

AHCA staff handled production of the *Here Are Your Choices* booklets. The RAND team provided them with camera-ready copy, prepared according to design decisions we made jointly and additional technical specifications they provided us. The booklets were included in the mailings to new Medicaid recipients in Volusia County during the months of November and December 1997. A supply of booklets also was made available to accompany the Decision Helper during its field test in the Daytona Beach welfare office.

DESIGN AND APPLICATION OF THE DECISION HELPER

The adaptation of the Decision Helper for a Medicaid population was performed during the summer 1997 with a targeted October 1 date to begin field testing the Medicaid Decision Helper in the Daytona Beach Economic Services Office. We describe here the decisions and activities involved in developing the Medicaid Decision Helper system and installing the system in the Economic Services Office. In approaching these tasks, the starting template we used for a Medicaid system was the CAHPS Decision Helper prototype that had been developed for the privately insured population. In doing so, we understood the need to modify the system to make it easier to use, and we viewed this demonstration as an opportunity to learn as much as possible about what features were necessary to achieve a feasible and effective system for Medicaid populations.

Between the time of our initial visits to the Daytona Beach and Ocala offices and final preparations for placing the Decision Helper in the field, there was a change in leadership in the Daytona Beach office. We were assured by the new Daytona Beach management team that they were prepared to proceed with the field test, and their management personnel fulfilled that commitment throughout subsequent working relationships. As discussed later in the report, however, the extent of this support was limited to a few individuals.

We entered the field expecting to find that not all Medicaid recipients would use the system — that the actual Decision Helper audience is a subset of the population who are comfortable using electronic information systems. Our goal was to learn who used the Decision Helper and why, and how might the system be made as "user friendly" as possible.

Adapting the Decision Helper Template to Florida Medicaid

As a first step in modifying the Decision Helper for use in the Florida Medicaid system, we demonstrated the CAHPS prototype Decision Helper with the Florida State staff of AHCA, Medicaid program, and Economic Services program. We did this by having them log on to the prototype version located on RAND's website. The participants gave us strong feedback that this system for the privately insured population needed to be simplified substantially for the Medicaid population, and they provided detailed comments on individual screens. The AHCA staff indicated they would be reluctant to move forward on the demonstration unless the Economic Services staff were comfortable with the Medicaid computer product. The following specific suggestions were offered for modifying the system:

- The language should be simple, at a 3rd-5th grade level if possible.
- The number of words (amount of information) on each screen should be reduced.
- The star charts are good and should be one of the first things the user sees. Users should be able to get to the chart with the global ratings from anywhere in the system.
- Bar charts appear useful but they are complex and may be hard to understand. The state staff felt that bars should not be used to report plan performance measures.
- The detailed survey statistics should not be provided for Medicaid beneficiaries.
- The feature "what's important to you" was well received, with no comment that it would be too complex for Medicaid users. They seemed comfortable with this amount of decision support and had no objections to summarizing reports and ratings of care to help users think through their decisions.
- Graphics should be added to point out the buttons that people should push to use the system.
- The path through the system should be made more linear so choices are simple and clear.
- The screens are too busy and should be simplified.
- Examples given on the consumer ratings page are too wordy, and some are not relevant to Medicaid recipients (e.g., many of them do not own cars).
- Medicaid users may never use a tutorial module in the system, so important training information (mouse training, icon definitions, how to get to charts, etc.) should be provided separately and early in their navigational path.
- Instructions for using the mouse should be the very first thing presented.
- A familiar symbol should be developed that can take users through the system.
- Give an initial screen that describes what each icon means, and use pop-ups on the icons to provide that information on every screen.
- The users should have print capability available, but it must be easy to use.

The State Economic Services staff made frequent references to using a kiosk style system, rather than a simple computer setup, and they stated their preference for a touch-screen system, both for ease of use and for equipment security. They warned that there are many children in the local service centers, and we should expect a mouse to "walk away" from an unsupervised system.

Given the feedback provided by the Florida state staff, we adopted a cornerstone criterion of "less is more" for designing a Decision Helper for the Florida Medicaid field test. We concluded that our first test with the Florida Medicaid population should field a simple system, and that more refinements could be added later, as we learned more about users' capabilities and preferences. This approach also was more feasible for software production with fixed resources.

A draft version of the Florida Medicaid Decision Helper was developed that incorporated many of the ideas generated by discussions with the Florida State staff. Not all their suggestions could be implemented because some differed from the goals of the Decision Helper or they were not feasible. For example, although we were able to lower the reading level of the text on the screens, it was not possible to achieve a 3rd to 5th grade level due to the inherent cognitive complexity of health care insurance concepts. The Decision Helper placed in the Daytona Beach Economic Services Office had the following features:

- Touch screen capability allowed users to navigate the system without a mouse.
- The path through the system was linear, with "next" and "back" buttons for navigation.
- Simple text was used on the computer screens, with few written words, large font, and 6th to 8th grade reading level.
- An animated host named Nina guided the user through the system and explained each screen.
- An introductory screen displayed a collage of graphics that fade in and out, including the Florida state seal and photographs of health care providers and consumers.
- Sound capability provided both background music for the introductory screen and Nina's voice.
- The comparative health plan ratings were limited to the "stars" and were displayed on two pages, one page for the global ratings and another for the composite reports.
- A search function was provided for users to find their physicians and identify the health plans in which the physicians participate.
- A decision support function assisted users in identifying the health plan features and ratings that are most important to them and summarizes plan performance on those dimensions.
- Users could print the information on the Decision Helper screens to take home with them.

Installing the Decision Helper in the Economic Services Office

With a goal of assessing the feasibility of using the Decision Helper for a Medicaid population, we planned the field test to minimize operational interventions by RAND during the test period, once we installed the system in the Economic Services Office. This approach allowed us to test the extent of support required for such a system and the willingness and capability of the local Economic Services Office to provide that support. We contracted with a local computer expert to provide technical support to the Economic Services staff for maintenance of the Decision Helper and troubleshooting system problems. This outside support simulated the capability that the Florida Medicaid program would provide if it were implementing the Decision Helper without RAND's involvement. We monitored the experiences of all parties involved with the system during the field test, including the local Economic Services staff who were our key contacts, other staff in the office, the clients in the office who chose to use (or not use) the Decision Helper, and the local technical support person with whom we contracted.

Design of the Decision Helper Console. When the State Medicaid and Economic Services staff reviewed the Decision Helper in preparation for the field test, they had expressed concern that people would not use the system unless special features were used to catch their attention. They suggested that we use a moving screen saver on the computer, use sound to advertise the system, place an eye-catching poster on the wall, and create a kiosk-style console by building a 3-dimensional backdrop that wraps around the computer so only the screen shows. As discussed above, we incorporated the first two suggestions into the design of the Medicaid Decision Helper. We also designed a large (3 feet x 4 feet) poster on which Nina invited people to use the Decision Helper and showed them how to start using it. We chose not to use a full kiosk design because we felt it was premature to invest substantially in such a system until the feasibility of the basic design had been field tested. Yet the console system we used was quite similar to a kiosk.

The choice of the physical form of the Decision Helper was guided by the requirements to get the attention of potential users, encourage their use of the system, and secure the equipment from theft or damage. The computer system was installed in a 5-foot tall metal cabinet with a lower closed compartment for the CPU and keyboard and a large top opening for the speakers and touch-screen monitor. The cabinet also had large, sturdy castors so it could be rolled out into its lobby location at the start of each day and rolled back into a closed room at the end of each day for security. The large castors were needed to get over the various thresholds on the system's path of movement. This cabinet was purchased and shipped to Daytona Beach in advance of the arrival of our field team for the Decision Helper installation.

On-Site Installation and Start-Up. Two members of RAND's CAHPS team managed all the preparation for the field test and the actual installation of the Decision Helper in the Daytona Beach office, working in collaboration with the management staff at the Daytona Beach office. RAND had responsibility for installation of the computer system, technical maintenance of the system, and removal of the system at the end of the field test for shipment back to RAND. These functions were performed by a combination of RAND staff and the local computer technician with whom we contracted to support the system. We asked the Economic Services Office to designate one staff person to turn the computer on and off each day, communicate with us when problems arose that required technical support, and perform other liaison functions.

RAND's field team took the following steps on-site in Daytona Beach for the installation of the Decision Helper in the local Economic Service office:

1. A walking tour of the site was performed to become familiar with the layout and meet the participating staff. Introductory folders were distributed containing information that included a overview of the project, a list of frequently asked questions, the RAND brochure, and brochures on RAND's health work.
2. As introductions were made to each staff group, the field team explained the process of how the implementation and evaluation would be done. They stressed that every key person involved in the field test know the contact information for the implementation and project teams, so we could be reached when they needed help.
3. The office layout was examined to identify options for Decision Helper location, routes of entry, stairs, locations of electrical outlets, and other installation requirements.
4. The cabinet and computer components were assembled and tested in the back section of the office. Although this area was out of the main flow of traffic, many people were curious and

visited the field team during setup, so the field team spent a good deal of time answering questions.

5. The printer was mounted permanently on top of the console by drilling up through the console and screwing metal screws into small holes in the printer's feet.

6. To address other security concerns raised by the reception area staff, the Decision Helper was locked at its location each day using a heavy-duty bicycle cable locked to an eye bolt in the floor. The staff were quite concerned that someone would roll the console out of the office if it were not secured.

7. Two local staff were designated as "technology maintainers" who had primary responsibility for rolling the Decision Helper into position each morning and back into the office at the end of each day. They also were responsible for recording problems with the computer and restarting the system when errors occurred. Our field team gave these individuals special training in the roll-out, boot-up, and shut-down procedures, supported by written documentation.

8. A triage system was worked out with the technology maintainers for handling problems with operation of the system. An inspection schedule was established where the technology maintainers checked on the Decision Helper at 2 to 3 hour intervals. If a problem was noticed, they would attempt to restart the system. If a client in the reception lobby reported a problem to the reception staff at the windows, these staff were instructed to alert one of the technology maintainers.

The RAND field team gave special attention to educating the general staff at the site to help them understand the technology, the field test purpose and approach, and arrangements made for local technical support for the Decision Helper. During preliminary preparations for the field test, we had unsuccessfully suggested having a formal training session for interested staff. Therefore, we used an informal training strategy instead. During the setup period our field team encouraged staff to ask questions and try out the system, and they emphasized that this was an experimental effort being done collaboratively with the local site and RAND. They also told the local office staff that RAND anticipated some problems with the system would occur, and that we hoped to learn from those experiences.

Making acceptable arrangements for the printer was one of the challenges faced by the field team. They originally had planned to place the printer on a table adjacent to the console. The Daytona Beach office staff vehemently disagreed with this plan, however, saying that children in the office lobby would quickly damage the printer by pulling paper from it, turning it on and off, and otherwise playing with it. After early observations confirmed this concern, the printer was bolted to the top of the cabinet. Computer and printer supplies were stored in the bottom of the cabinet, including a box of paper for the printer. Although the paper supply provided balancing weight for the slightly top-heavy console, this extra weight also made the console hard to roll and difficult to get back through doorway to the overnight storage site.

Section 3

EVALUATION METHODS AND DATA

To evaluate the field tests of the Florida Medicaid paper report format and Decision Helper, we wanted to obtain information from the major stakeholders involved in use of these reports. AHCA and the Medicaid program were obvious stakeholders, as sponsors of the survey and consumer reports. Others included Medicaid recipients who would use these reports and Medicaid health plans whose performances were being compared. In addition, the state and local Economic Services Offices were important stakeholders for field placements of the Decision Helper in local Economic Services Offices. As discussed above, if the Decision Helper was to become a part of the Medicaid information activities, these offices would be the likely locations to house them.

In this section, we describe methods that we used to undertake three major evaluation tasks designed to obtain feedback from representatives of each of these major stakeholders, seeking to learn as much as possible from their differing perspectives:

- Obtain consumer feedback on the paper report by conducting two focus groups with Medicaid recipients in January 1998.

- Evaluation of the Decision Helper field test in the Daytona Beach Economic Services office, including observations of use of the system, exit interviews of users, and analysis of daily use logs generated by the Decision Helper software.

- Performance of a 2-day site visit to Florida to conduct individual and group interviews about both reporting media, after field tests of the paper report and Decision Helper were completed; interviewing representatives of AHCA, the Medicaid program, Economic Services Offices, the MediPass program, and the two HMOs serving Volusia County.

FOCUS GROUP EVALUATION OF THE PAPER REPORTS

To obtain consumer feedback on the *Here Are Your Choices* booklet, two focus groups were conducted on January 24, 1998 in a local library in Daytona Beach. Groups were led by a single moderator, and one observer from the State was present for both groups. A copy of the topic guide used for the focus groups is in Appendix C. Group participants were asked to review and comment on the *Here Are Your Choices* booklet. They also were asked to provide feedback on alternative page formats for displaying the stars for comparative health plan performance, which are in Appendix D.

All participants were recruited by RAND using Volusia County Medicaid enrollment lists covering November and December 1997, all of whom had been mailed the *Here Are Your Choices* report. The lists included AFDC and SSI populations. To be candidates for the focus groups, an individual had to enroll themselves or their children in Medicaid during November or December 1997, be age 18 or older, and be on Medicaid or the parent or guardian of a child on Medicaid.

Two focus groups were conducted, each with 10 participants. Demographic data on the participants were collected in a brief background questionnaire completed by each participant before the focus group began. The questionnaire was voluntary and anonymous. The characteristics of the participants are summarized in Table 2. Half the participants remembered receiving the consumer report. Seven of the 20 group participants reported that they chose a plan. Four of these seven participants reported using the consumer report to choose a plan.

Table 2
Characteristics of Florida Medicaid Focus Group Participants

Participant Characteristics	Number of Participants	Participant Characteristics	Number of Participants
Total participants	20		
Mean number of children <age 18*	2.7	**Family Medicaid Profile:**	
		Participant enrolled	10
Gender:		One or more children enrolled	18
Male	1	Other family members enrolled	1
Female	19		
		Medicaid Plan:**	
Education:		MediPass	13
8th grade or less	2	PCA Family Health Plan	4
Some high school	5	United HealthCare of Florida, Inc.	1
GED or high school diploma	6	Other (FFS Medicaid)	1
Vocational school or some college	3	No data	2
College degree	3		
Professional or graduate degree	0		
No data	1	**CAHPS Report Booklet:**	
		Remember getting it	10
Marital status:		Used it to choose plan	4
Currently married	8		
Not married	12	**Plan Selection:**	
		Assigned a plan	12
Race/Ethnicity:		Chose a plan	7
African American or Black	11	No data	1
Hispanic or Latino	0		
Native American/American Indian	1		
Asian and Pacific Islander	1		
White	7		
Other	0		

*   includes grandchildren for whom participant is legal guardian

**   Total exceeds number of participants because one person reported two grandchildren in different plans (MediPass and PCA)

EVALUATION OF THE DECISION HELPER

Multiple methods were used to evaluate the performance of the Florida Medicaid Decision Helper, including both qualitative and quantitative techniques. This diversity of methods reflects the complexity of factors and participants involved in establishing and maintaining such a system in a local setting. The information collected through the individual evaluation techniques was compared and synthesized to achieve a cohesive set of field test findings.

The primary focus of the evaluation was to learn from the experiences of the individuals who used the Daytona Beach economic services office during the time the Decision Helper was in operation. We were interested in documenting the frequency of use for the Decision Helper, reasons why people did or did not use it, the extent to which they looked at the information it provided, and their assessments of how easy it was to use and the value of the information. A combination of observation techniques, exit interviews, and computer logs were used to collect this information. We performed observations of Decision Helper use and conducted exit interviews during the first six business days of November. We chose this time period because the first week of each month is the busiest time for the economic services office, so we could obtain sufficient sample size for analysis from a limited number of days in the field.

In addition to the potential users, we also wanted to document the experiences with the Decision Helper of the various parties involved in operating the field test. As discussed in Section 1, a local Economic Services Office is the best candidate as the location for the Decision Helper because it is the only physical facility at which contact is made with Medicaid recipients, yet the field test is being sponsored by the state Medicaid office. The feasibility of a broader application of the Decision Helper will depend on the experiences and perspectives of both organizations in this field test.

Notes of RAND Field Team

As described above, two RAND team members were on-site in Daytona Beach to install the Decision Helper in the Economic Services Office. They prepared detailed field notes to document the events that occurred during the installation process, reactions from the Economic Services Office staff and clients, arrangements forged with the local technical support person, and other issues that they faced in getting the Decision Helper operational. These field notes captured our initial insights regarding an array of implementation issues that will be faced by any sponsor using such a computer-based system to provide consumers comparative health plan information. In our process evaluation analysis, we summarized the key lessons learned from the field notes and considered their implications as part of our synthesis of findings from the various evaluation components.

Computer Logs

Throughout the time the Decision Helper was operating in the Daytona Beach office, an internal computer log collected detailed data on every encounter with the system. The log recorded the time when a user began a session, what screens were used, and how long the user remained on each screen. It also noted when sessions were terminated because of periods of inactivity, with return to the introductory screen. The local technical support person downloaded the log contents periodically during the field test period and transmitted the data to RAND technical staff.

The log data provided valuable information on the full scope of use of the Decision Helper during normal periods of operation when no evaluation interventions were being performed. We analyzed the data to learn the extent to which the Decision Helper was used and which aspects of the system were used most frequently. Descriptive summaries were prepared of the number of sessions, the lengths of sessions, the pages at which sessions terminated, and the amounts of time spent on each page.

Observations of Decision Helper Activity

At the end of the month of field placement, we performed structured observations of the extent to which customers of the economic services office used the Decision Helper. An observation form was prepared delineating the observation data to be collected, which is provided in Appendix E. The observation information collected included:

- demographic characteristics of each potential user,
- whether the person was alone or accompanied by others (children or adults),
- whether and how long the person actually used the Decision Helper, and
- whether the person used the printer.

Two data collectors were sent to the Daytona Beach economic services office to perform the observation task on Monday and Tuesday, November 3 and 4, 1997. They completed an observation form for each adult individual who approached the Decision Helper and remained in front of it for at least 5 seconds (qualified individuals). They also counted the total number of adults who entered the economic services office, to obtain a denominator for estimating overall Decision Helper use rates. Observation data were collected before the exit interviews to ensure that the observations accurately reflected "steady state" Decision Helper usage, recognizing that performing the interviews would disrupt usage patterns.

Exit Interviews in the Economic Services Office

The exit interviews were personal interviews designed to obtain feedback from potential users of the Decision Helper regarding the system itself, factors that contributed to their decisions to use the Decision Helper or not, their perceptions of the features of the system, and their views regarding the usefulness of the information it provides. Anyone who approached the Decision Helper and examined the first page for at least a brief period (15 seconds) was included in the survey sample because we were seeking feedback from those who chose not to use the system as well as those who used it. Individuals were interviewed immediately after they approached or used the Decision Helper. The interviews were conducted on November 5, 6, 7, and 10, 1997, by the same data collectors who performed the observations of Decision Helper activity on the previous two days. Each respondent was paid $5 for completing the interview.

The exit interview was limited to 5 minutes or less in length to encourage good response rates. We used two interview forms, both of which contained a common set of 12 questions that were asked of all qualified individuals plus another 11 questions that were asked only of those who used the Decision Helper. In addition, each form contained 5 questions that were not on the other form. This two-form approach allowed us to ask a larger number of questions than could be accommodated on one questionnaire within the time limit we imposed. The questionnaire forms are in Appendix F.

All individuals interviewed were asked about their previous experience using a computer or similar system, what led them to approach the Decision Helper, their perceptions of the system and the information it contains, and the timeliness of the information provided by the Decision Helper for their Medicaid plan decisions. Respondents also were asked what information the Economic Services staff gave them, including any information about Medicaid, choosing a health plan, or using the computer system to help choice. Background information was collected on respondent demographics and prior experience with welfare, Medicaid, or Medicaid health plans.

Individuals who actually used the computer were asked additional questions on their reactions to using the Decision Helper, the importance of having a paper printout to take home, their comfort with using the computer as a stand-alone system with no assistance, and whether they would use the Decision Helper again.

Word-of-mouth information about the exit interview payments led to the participation of motorcyclists (bikers), homeless persons, and others who might not otherwise have entered the economic services office. The interviewers coded these individuals whenever they could identify them, for consideration during analysis. A total of 185 exit interviews were completed, about 40 percent of whom were not current users of the economic services office. Although the characteristics of these other users differed somewhat from the target Medicaid population, many either had been or were eligible to be Medicaid recipients. We concluded that they represented a potential Medicaid population and their reactions to the Decision Helper provided useful information for the field test.

PROCESS EVALUATION SITE VISIT AND INTERVIEWS

A site visit to Florida was conducted by two RAND team members on December 17 and 18, 1997, during which they interviewed 15 individuals in AHCA, the State Economic Services Office, and the Daytona Beach office where the Decision Helper was field tested. The purpose of the interviews was to learn from these demonstration participants about which aspects of the CAHPS report formats were useful, where we might improve the products, and what implementation issues must be managed when using the products in the field. The evaluation information was intended to provide feedback for strengthening the CAHPS report products and implementation guide, to help make them more effective for subsequent CAHPS sponsors. We worked with the process evaluation protocol and interview guide developed by the CAHPS consortium evaluation team, adapting them to address the field testing of report formats in the Florida Medicaid demonstration. A copy of the interview guide used for this evaluation is presented in Appendix G.

With the goal of obtaining a good mix of perspectives regarding the paper report and Decision Helper, we interviewed a variety of individuals who were relevant to the field test. The first day of the site visit was spent in Daytona Beach, interviewing key individuals involved in the Decision Helper field test. We interviewed the two Economic Services Office staff who worked with RAND to install the Decision Helper and provided the daily system support during the field test. We also talked with the local technical person with whom we had contracted to provide technical assistance for problems that could not be resolved by a simple re-boot of the system. On the second day, we went to Tallahassee to interview key leadership staff from AHCA, the director of the Medicaid managed care program, lead staff in the MediPass program, and the state-level Economic Services staff. During that day, we also conducted a telephone interview with representatives of the two health plans serving Medicaid recipients in Volusia County.

EVALUATION FINDINGS FOR THE PAPER REPORT

During the demonstration, the AHCA, Medicaid, and Economic Services staff expressed a number of views about what would be needed to make the paper report useful for new Medicaid recipients, which drew upon their years of experience working with their clients. Yet such field experience often yields anecdotal information, which may not fully represent the information needs of the entire population. This demonstration offered us an opportunity to test some of these design issues empirically, and thereby strengthen the factual basis for design decisions by both our Florida collaborators and ourselves.

Given the diversity of human information requirements and display preferences, we felt it was important to synthesize evaluation information from various perspectives regarding the design of the written report, *Here Are Your Choices*. Therefore, we used a combination of focus groups with Medicaid recipients and interviews with state agency staff as our information sources for the evaluation of the report document. This Section presents the results of this evaluation. First we discuss the results of the two focus groups that we conducted in January 1998, and then we summarize findings from the site visit interviews regarding the strengths and weaknesses of the paper report.

FOCUS GROUP RESULTS

General Findings

The Enrollment Process. Participants expressed frustration with the Medicaid health plan enrollment process. Despite County assurances that all newly eligible Medicaid recipients were mailed information packets describing Medicaid benefits and the enrollment process, many participants reported that they never received an information packet. As one participant expressed it, "I went and signed my son up and the next thing I got was a card in the mail telling me who his doctor and plan are." Another participant said "I didn't get any paperwork [from the County]." Participants in one focus group felt that regular US Mail was not a good way to deliver materials to them. They reported that they often don't see mail addressed to them because others in the household (such as teenage children) may open the household's mail first. Participants in both groups report that the mail is not secure in their neighborhood, or mail delivery is not reliable. Group participants felt that they would be more likely to actually receive mail that required their signature. Quite a few reported that they felt the only reason our Federal Express packet confirming their invitation to the group reached them was because they had to sign for it.

When to Provide the Consumer Report. Virtually all participants felt the consumer report should be given to you when you go to sign up for Medicaid. They felt that it was better to make a choice before eligibility is determined and get that choice "entered into the computer" so that if you (or your child) are indeed eligible, the plan you picked is already recorded in the system. This response implies that, for at least some individuals, early availability of health plan information is desirable rather than premature. In a somewhat contradictory finding, all participants wanted to have a telephone number to call to ask more questions and get more information. In general, participants felt it was important to have the consumer hotline number printed on the report, and they would call it. One participant said she would not use consumer data at all, but instead would call the hotline and ask questions to get the information she needed to choose among the available plans. A few participants thought that a [welfare] caseworker should give them the report and review it with them, explaining the contents and how to use it. "I would like to be able to, first of all, choose, you know HMO and MediPass and have [the difference] explained to you. That way you'll be able to talk with somebody about it and if you have any questions, ask questions."

While 10 people indicated in the background questionnaire that they had received the consumer report, only 4 people in the group thought the report looked familiar. No one verbally reported that they had used the booklet to choose a plan, although the one participant who had not yet chosen a plan took her materials home and was going to make a choice. This finding contradicts the background questionnaire data in which 4 individuals reported using the booklet to choose a plan. Collectively, these results suggest that many people have trouble distinguishing the contents of the information materials they are provided.

Reactions to the Report Booklet

Almost everyone in both focus groups understood the concept of the stars in the "star report." Both groups spent considerable time looking through the report, and overall, the participants accurately reported what it meant for a health plan to have one, two, or three stars. One participant was confused by the stars, thinking that the number of stars was tied in to the number of plans, and that one star meant the plan was the lowest of the three in the given composite and three stars meant it was the best. Another participant commented that most of us think in terms of 4 star ratings as being the best (4 star hotel, 4 star restaurant). She wondered why 4 stars were not set up as the best, with stars then taken away based on reports from people who used the plan.

Participants in both focus groups discussed what it meant when all the plans were "average," which was the case for the global ratings for plans serving Volusia County (on page 4 of the report). Specific comments about the global plan star ratings reflected the absence of differences among the plans:

> » "Everything's average all right."
> » "All these [plans] are not the same but they're listed as the same."
> » "You might as well just close your eyes and pick one."
> » "If you look at this, you know, looking at the stars it looks like one is just as good as another."

Trust in the ratings. Although the focus group participants felt, in general, that consumer ratings were helpful, some participants (especially those in group 2) were distrustful of the ratings. One participant said that she thought her standards were higher than other people's standards, so she deducted 1 star from each composite (basically downgrading or weighting the ratings). Early in the focus group session, some participants said the report "reads like a sales pitch for MediPass" and "Did MediPass put out this [report]?" These comments may argue for placing the explanation of the survey and data collection closer to the front of the report (it was at the end of the Florida Medicaid report). Quite a few participants said they would also seek information from other sources, and they would try to find someone enrolled in a plan to talk with about their experience with the plan.

The two focus groups differed in the reasons given for not trusting the ratings. Group 1 participants were more willing to trust a "below average" rating than an "above average" rating as it seemed more honest to them. Plan reports that did not match an individual's experience with a particular plan (or the experience of a friend or family member) were distrusted. General consensus from the group 2 participants who expressed a lack of trust in the ratings was that people's opinions differ, so that reports from others would not tell them what a health plan would be like for them. With participants for both focus groups recruited the same way, the differences in their responses simply reflects diversity in individual perceptions of the ratings, with the more vocal people in each group having differing views.

Reference to survey sample. Some participants did not like the sentence on page 4 (star page) that refers to "people like you." One participant asked "Who are people like me? Are they on Medicaid? Do they have kids? Where do they live?" Another said that "people like you" sounds negative and "like a put down." Other comments included:

» "It makes me feel like 'us poor people'."
» "I think it could have been worded better."
» "I'm sorry, some of us come from different backgrounds. Maybe that worked for them but it's not gonna work for me."
» "Who <u>are</u> the people they choose to do the survey?"

Information about the survey. As mentioned above, participants wanted to see the description of the survey earlier in the report. In fact, this became an issue for some people by the time they reached page 2. Participants wanted to know if the ratings came only from people in Medicaid or from everyone in the HMO plans. Did they survey everyone in Florida? Everyone in the county? Specific reactions to the last page, which describes the survey and how it was conducted, were:

• A total of 939 responses was not thought to be enough to be representative, and a 38 percent response rate meant that "hardly anyone" answered the survey.

• Participants wanted to know if people got money for answering the survey, expressing concern that a financial incentive might cause respondents to give more favorable reports of the plan.

• There were concerns that the survey vendor did not try to reach some people by telephone because not everyone gets their mail (as discussed above).

• Participants felt that six months of enrollment is not enough time to know a plan.

• Participants wanted to know about the amount and type of experience and number of visits of the people who answered the survey.

• There was a desire to know what people who have children with serious health conditions think about the plans. An individual with a specific condition (in this case, diabetes) wanted to know if separate ratings could be reported for survey respondents with that condition.

• With knowledge that health plans did not sponsor the survey or produce the report, participants perceived that the information in the report was more reliable than they originally thought.

- Participants emphasized that people who have had problems with their health plans should be included in the survey, to be sure that information is collected from people who really know what a plan is like.

Additional plan information. When probed to identify additional information they felt the plan member survey should collect, participants listed the following:

- How the survey respondents got on Medicaid (participants felt that this information would help them decide the extent to which survey respondents were like them);
- Reports of the types of problems that people had with their plans.

Making report more useful. When probed to identify information that would make the reports more useful, participants listed the following:

- Detailed information on benefits and coverage, including which prescriptions are covered or not, what co-pays are for each plan, what procedures are required for an ER visit;
- Detailed information on dental care covered benefits and provider locations;
- A list of the doctors participating with each plan and their office locations;
- The locations of hospitals and emergency rooms participating with each plan;
- The locations of facilities for laboratory tests, if different from the doctor's office or clinic;
- A list of specialists participating in the plan and their locations (some participants have found that, for some specialties, no specialist in Daytona Beach accepts Medicaid);
- Information on which procedures require prior authorization from the plan;
- Information on what is required to get a referral to a specialist from the primary care doctor;
- A description of each plan's complaint process, and how long it takes for a complaint to be resolved.

Group participants did not have extensive comments about the "tip boxes" found in the report, although they felt they were useful and should stay in report. The tip on page 8, which said that each family member could choose a different provider, was identified by a show of hands as the most useful tip. One participant noted that the tip box on page 7 (about enrollees in Children's Medical Services having to choose MediPass) gave information she had tried unsuccessfully to get from the local Medicaid office.

One participant, in particular, felt the report would be more useful if it caught the reader's attention, saying. "I don't want to hurt your feelings, but this is bo-ring. Can't you use color or pictures to make it more exciting?" It was not clear how prevalent this sentiment was among participants.

Alternative Report Formats

The focus groups took some time to review two alternative formats for presenting the plan ratings. The goal was to compare the alternative formats to each other, and to the format used in the *Here Are Your Choices* booklet. The alternative versions were (see Appendix D):

- dimension by dimension format (one composite per page, shown for all plans),
- matrix format (all plans and report categories together on a single page).

The two focus groups differed in their format preferences. In general, group 1 favored the dimension by dimension format (all plans on one page, one composite per page). However, the reason for this preference was because it was the only format where they noticed that phone numbers were printed for the plans. They felt the increase in number of pages was acceptable because the information would be easier to read than the current format of one plan per page (pages 6-8 in the report). Participants in this group believed strongly that "simpler is better" and they felt that the dimension-by-dimension report met that criterion. Group 2 (8 out of 10 participants) favored the matrix format over the dimension-by-dimension format, because they preferred to see all the plans on one page. The majority of the group 2 participants felt that the matrix format should replace pages 6-8 in the current report. However, at least one respondent in group 2 reported that the booklet should contain both the current single-plan per page format and an additional page in the matrix format. It is difficult to explore such issues in any detail in a focus group format, and the issues raised in these discussions merit further follow-up with cognitive interviews or some other one-on-one interview method.

FEEDBACK FROM SITE VISIT INTERVIEWS

Strengths of written report

The AHCA and State Medicaid staff reported that they believed the star counts are easy to grasp visually. The stars are effective as symbols to compare one health plan's performance to the others offer, where two stars represent average performance for the plans serving the county. The stars also serve as a type of graph, where a longer horizontal graph (3 stars) is better than a short one (1 star), thus helping users see the information easily.

The other report feature appreciated by the State staff were the "step-by-step" directions provided for how to use the booklet and how to choose a health plan. They believed these features could be quite useful as they refine their enrollment counseling activities.

Criticisms of written report

As discussed in Section 2, the *Here Are Your Choices* booklet was folded in half so it would fit into the envelope that Florida uses to Medicaid mail enrollment materials. Although the booklet looked like a book, it actually opened to pages that were in landscape format on 8 ½" x 11" paper with printing on both sides. These pages were fastened by one staple in the top left corner (when opened). The large, folded pages were difficult and awkward to handle, and it was especially difficult to flip over the pages to read the reverse sides.

The summary chart that showed the global ratings for each of the three health plan choices had two stars in all six cells of the chart—the plans did not differ on these ratings. Thus, this chart did not help Medicaid recipients to choose a health plan, and it may have discouraged recipients from reading any further to look at the more detailed reports on specific dimensions of performance by plan, where there were some differences in plan performance.

The Medicaid office did not use a photograph supplied by RAND for the cover (a picture of an Asian child) because it was not "racially neutral" and it was not consistent with the demographics of Volusia County, where there are relative few Asians. Instead, the state substituted a less visually interesting, but uncontroversial picture of the state seal.

The State staff felt that side-by-side comparisons of the plans were more helpful in revealing differences among plans than the plan-by-plan pages that the report used. However, a layout that revealed marked differences among plans might have been less politically acceptable to both the plans and the state officials responsible for the quality of care provided to Medicaid recipients. The following specific issues were raised regarding the presentation and layout of the report:

- The report layout was too busy. The pages with the plan-specific star ratings also included a large checkbox and a "tip" box, which competed with the ratings for attention.
- The report was too wordy, and there was too little white space on each page.
- Because the report presented each health plan's star ratings on a separate page, it would have been too long if there had been more than three plan choices.

There was consensus that developing the *Here Are Your Choices* booklet for one county was not really a fair test of what statewide implementation would entail. If separate county reports were published, it would have been much more difficult and costly for the state to prepare and mail materials for recipients in all 67 Florida counties. The state currently develops a single, statewide "choice guide" that is relatively general, because it is too difficult and expensive to compile current, accurate information (such as phone numbers for plans) that is specific to each county. Most likely they would use a similar format for the health plan ratings report.

Section 5

FINDINGS FROM THE DECISION HELPER FIELD TEST

The purpose of the Florida field test of the Medicaid Decision Helper was to obtain empirical information regarding the required conditions for successful implementation of a decision-making support tool for a Medicaid population. Information obtained from this demonstration guided further development of the Decision Helper for subsequent testing in the New Jersey Medicaid program. Specific goals of the field test were to:

- Examine the acceptability to the Florida Medicaid population of the information provided in the Decision Helper;
- Identify and test the features required to make the system easy to use for Medicaid recipients;
- Identify the required administrative, physical, and logistical conditions that facilitate use of the Decision Helper in the field.

In this Section, we present evaluation results from the Daytona Beach field test of the Decision Helper. We first summarize issues that arose during the field installation of the Decision Helper and implications for future applications. They we present summary data on the utilization activity of the system, which was collected from computer logs and field observations. Results of our exit interviews then are presented, including findings about the extent of use of the system by low income consumers, their perceptions of the usability of the system, and their feedback on the usefulness of the health plan ratings. Finally, we summarize results of interviews with staff of the state and local agencies involved in the field test regarding the strengths and weaknesses of the Decision Helper. Implications are discussed for use of computer-based media to report comparative rating information to consumers.

In our original concept of the Decision Helper field test, we expected that some ongoing staff support would be provided to help recipients use the computer-based system. It quickly became clear that the Florida Economic Services Offices did not have the staff resources to provide such support. AHCA initially considered installing a telephone with the Medicaid 800 number at the Decision Helper location, but ultimately concluded that a telephone line would not be feasible. As a result, this demonstration tested the Decision Helper operating under what we viewed as "worst case" conditions as a completely independent system offered passively to potential users.

RESULTS OF THE DAYTONA BEACH FIELD TEST

Issues Identified During Field Installation

It did not take long to begin learning from our field test. The field notes prepared by our field team that installed the Decision Helper in Daytona Beach documented several issues that arose during the installation process. We summarize here several highlights of these early findings.

Efficiency of system and printer. Operating problems with both the computer and printer created barriers that reduced users' access to the Decision Helper's full capability. The system itself operated slowly on some screens, especially in the section where users searched for their physicians. In addition, three problems were identified with the printer: printer speed, need for instructions on the screen, ability to print multiple copies. The printer took about 1.5 minutes to print out a typical page. Although the user can continue navigating the screens during printing (the software spooled to the printer), this information was not given to the users, and printing had the potential to be a significant bottleneck. We concluded that the printer should be a fairly high speed variety (e.g. 5-6 page per minute) to reduce delays, which would increase the cost of a fully equipped Decision Helper. In addition, the software should display an explicit acknowledgment of the user's print request, and it should set a maximum on the number of repeated print requests on the same page. In a number of sessions, large numbers of copies were printed, apparently because of repetitive touches on the "print" button. Causes of this problem could be re-entering of print requests because users did not know the requests were being processed, or simply people playing with the printer. There also should be a feature to flush the print queue easily when restarting the software.

How to configure the physical work space. System design inevitably has implications for the container of the system itself, choice of location in the office, work space for the users, and associated requirements for chairs and other furniture. The system we had designed for this field test was one that allowed for some time and thinking as users consider their health plan choices. This design differs from the typical kiosk, which is intended for a more limited (3 to 5 minute) session. As discussed in Section 2, we chose a console-type physical structure for the system to accommodate a variety of user, security, and logistical considerations. We learned quickly, however, that the basic configuration of the lobby area in which the console was located placed constraints on our ability to achieve the desired configuration. The lobby layout influenced how chairs, table, or other furniture can be used to support the system. These issues need to be anticipated during preparation for a field placement of such a system.

Security of equipment. We arrived in the field believing we were well aware of the security issues to be faced during the field test, but we discovered that we had under-estimated the importance of security provisions. In this unsupervised lobby area, we learned from both the office staff and clients that anything mobile -- from the computer itself to the printer and paper -- was at risk of being stolen or vandalized. Thus, extra security provisions were undertaken in the field to reduce the risk of loss. These provisions were successful, in that all of the system components were still present and intact at the end of the field test period.

Requirements for daily maintenance and support. The importance of daily maintenance to a successful Decision Helper field placement cannot be over-stated. Yet this aspect of implementation could be overlooked because of the many other issues competing for the installers' attention. We identified four elements that must be addressed to ensure adequate maintenance for the system.

1. The leadership of the local office must have a clear commitment to ensuring that the Decision Helper system is managed effectively.

2. Orientation to the Decision Helper and training in its use need to be provided to local office staff so they are comfortable working with it.

3. A few office staff need to be given responsibility to provide the daily support for the system, including checking periodically during the day that the system is operating properly.

4. External technical support needs to be made available locally to troubleshoot problems that are beyond the ability of the office staff to manage.

Getting people's attention. The advice offered by the Florida State Economic Services staff about getting the attention of potential users was absolutely correct. To draw people's attention and guide them to touch the screen, we used a combination of a large poster, a moving collage of graphics on the introductory screen of the Decision Helper system, background music, and an array of signs posted on the computer. Even with this highly visible array of features, people were reluctant to use the system, and those who did approach it often were confused about how to start working with it. In retrospect, we concluded that displaying "Just touch the screen to start" in a large letters on the first screen might have helped potential users.

Ease of navigating the system. Some navigational barriers were identified immediately after the Decision Helper was placed in the Daytona Beach office. A check list box displayed on the top left corner of each screen was mis-interpreted by many users. This box was intended to show users where they were in the system, but many people tried to use the box as a menu to move from one section of the system to another. They often did not see the "next" and "back" arrows located on the bottom of the screen. Several people told our field team that they were interested in only one aspect of the information in the Decision Helper, and they were frustrated that they had to move linearly all the way through the system to reach that location. They wanted a menu capability that, in fact, we had not provided for the sake of simplicity.

Activity Patterns Identified in Computer Logs

A total of 229 sessions were recorded in the Decision Helper computer log over a total of 9 business days that the system operated routinely in the Daytona Beach office, for an average of 25.4 sessions per day. The actual volume of use ranged from 2 to 47 sessions daily. In Figure 1, we show the distribution of sessions by how many of the screens the users saw when they used the system. Over 70 of the 229 sessions did not go beyond the first screen that introduced the Decision Helper. Three-quarters of the sessions used 4 or fewer screens and over 90 percent used 7 or fewer screens, although almost 20 sessions moved through 13 screens. Screen 7 describes the extra benefits covered by the health plans available to Medicaid recipients in Volusia County, and screen 13 is the second page of consumer ratings for these health plan options. Only 10 sessions went through all 17 of the screens in the entire system.

For the Decision Helper sessions that went beyond the introductory screen (i.e., that actually used the system), people used the system for an average of 3.1 minutes. However, the amount of time varied widely from 1 to 31 minutes with a median of 2 minutes, as shown in Figures 2 and 3. The preponderance of short-length sessions reflect the small number of screens reached by most sessions, as shown in Figure 2. We also tabulated how frequently Decision Helper users printed pages with information to take home with them. The printer was used during 19.9 percent of the sessions, and for those sessions, the users printed an average of 1.5 pages per session.

The amount of time spent on each Decision Helper screen that users reached was estimated from the log data. The system is programmed to "time out" a session after a page remained on the screen for 35 minutes. Therefore, for the last page of a session, we were not able to determine how much of the time was spent by a user looking actively at the page and how much was dead time after the user had left the Decision Helper. As a result, the times we calculated over-estimate usage of screens to some extent, but they still provide comparative information on variations in screen usage. Indeed, we found that the average time varied substantially depending on the type of information being provided on the screens.

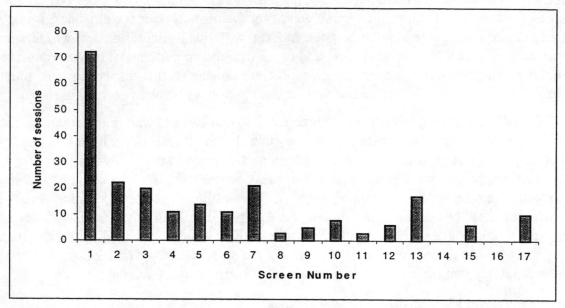

Figure 1. Distribution of Decision Helper Sessions by Number of Screens Used

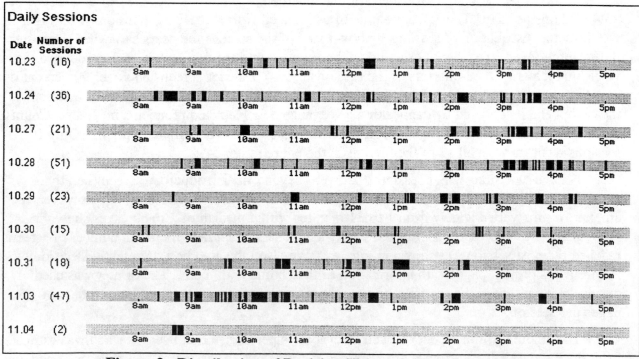

Figure 2. Distribution of Decision Helper Sessions Over Time

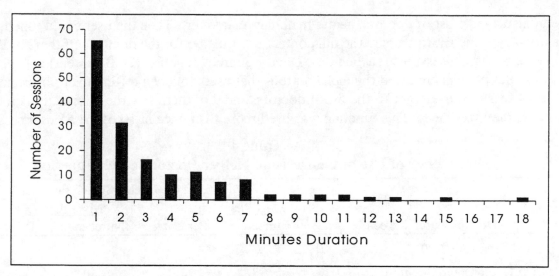

Figure 3. Duration of Decision Helper Sessions That Exceeded One Screen

As shown in Table 3, users spent the longest time looking at the screens with the consumer rating information and the screens that helped them find the health plans with which their physicians were affiliated. Somewhat less time was spent using screens that describe the health plan benefits, and the least time was spent on the introductory screens that greet the user and provide definitions of Medicaid and the plan choices that beneficiaries need to make.

Table 3
Estimated Average Time Spent on Each Screen for Users Who Reached the Screen

Decision Helper Screen	Average Number of Minutes	Decision Helper Screen	Average Number of Minutes
Average for all screens	2.08		
Rating of plan features	12.40	Primary care provider intro	2.97
Summary of plan ratings	8.80	List of extra benefits	2.10
Summary of results for plans	8.47	List of basic benefits	1.49
		Compare HMO & Medipass	1.25
Plan ratings with user priorities	5.82		
Alphabet key to find doctor	5.43	Medicaid plan choices	0.89
Print doctor information	5.14	Introduction	0.58
Consumer rating PF	4.97	What Is Medicaid	0.55
Select from listed doctors	4.84		
Definitions of rating dimensions	3.98		
Consumer rating introduction	3.79		
Introduce provider search	3.62		

The pattern of use of the "Doctor Search" function is presented in Table 4. This function used an alphabet tool to help users find out the health plans affiliations for specific physicians. When a user touched the first letter of the last name of the doctor on the alphabet tool, the next screen displayed a list of doctors' names matching that letter. Then the user could touch the name of a doctor on the list to display the full contact information for the doctor. Of the 229 Decision Helper sessions, 55 sessions reached the "Doctor Search" function (24.0 percent) and 19 of those sessions (8.3 percent) reached the alpha buttons that users touched to find their physicians. In 14 of the 19 sessions, users got to the list of doctors, and 9 of them saw the information on the physician they specified. This function was used more than once in 10 of the 55 user sessions.

Table 4
Frequency of Use of the Decision Helper Doctor Search Function

| | Saw Pages in the Doctor Search Function | | | |
| | At Least Once | | More than Once | |
Doctor Search Screen	Number	Percent	Number	Percent
Total sessions = 229				
Saw Doctor Search button	55	24.0	10	4.4
Entered Doctor Search:				
Got to Alpha buttons	19	8.3	6	2.6
Got to list of doctors	14	6.1	4	1.7
Information on specific doctor	9	3.9	3	1.3

Observed Usage of the Decision Helper

During two days of observation, a total of 54 adults met our "approach" criterion of spending at least 15 seconds looking at the Decision Helper. These persons represented 8.4 percent of the 640 adults who we counted entering the Daytona Beach economic services office during the observation period. As shown in Table 5, over two-thirds of the adults who approached the Decision Helper were female. About 39 percent of the potential users (approachers) were African American, 44 percent were white, and 14 percent were Hispanic or Latino. We were not able to compare this group of Decision Helper users to the larger population because we did not have demographic data for the overall customer mix of the Economic Services Office, nor did we collect such data for all people entering the office during the observation days.

Summary profile information on observed use of the Decision Helper during the two days of observation is reported in Table 6. Over 60 percent of individuals were alone when they used the Decision Helper, 27 percent were accompanied by one or more other adults, and almost 12 percent had children with them. Almost half of the individuals used the Decision Helper for less than a minute, and slightly more than 21 percent used it for greater than 5 minutes.

These observation results are consistent with the distribution of sessions recorded by the computer log for usage prior to the evaluation. More than 63 percent of the 5-minute (or more) users printed out health plan information from their sessions, in contrast to much lower percentages of the shorter-term users. The small sample of observed users limited our ability to detect statistically significant differences in use patterns by users' characteristics. However, differences between males and females were close to significant for both time of use and whether they used the printer to print out pages of results, with females tending to spend more time at the computer and to be more likely to use the printer. With a larger sample, we might be able to infer that significant differences do exist for these items.

Table 5
Demographics of Adults Who Approached the
Decision Helper During the Observation Period

Characteristic	Percentage
Gender	
Female	69.2
Male	30.8
Race/ethnicity	
African American	38.5
Hispanic/Latino	13.5
White	44.2
Asian	1.9
Other	1.9

Table 6
Use of the Decision Helper During the Observation Period

Aspects of Use	Percentage
Situation	
Was alone	61.5
With non-participating children	3.9
With participating children	7.7
With non-participating adults	11.5
With participating adults	15.4
Time of use	
Less than 1 minute	48.1
1 to 5 minutes	30.8
More than 5 minutes	21.2
Used printer, by time of use	
Less than 1 minute	0***
1 to 5 minutes	12.5***
More than 5 minutes	63.4***

*** $p < 0.001$

Exit Interviews

As discussed in the Methods section, we paid $5 to each individual who participated in the exit interview, to include at least some consideration of the Decision Helper and completion of the full exit interview. These payments led to participation in the field test by many individuals who would not otherwise have been in the Economic Services office. With an interest in understanding how these respondents may have affected our evaluation results, we began our analysis of the exit interview data by comparing responses obtained from the Economic Services Office users ("target group") to those obtained from other individuals ("outside users"). As shown in Table 7, the two groups differed in gender and Medicaid status. Almost two-thirds of the target group were female, whereas the outside group was predominantly male. The racial/ethnic mix of the two groups was similar. Slightly more than half of the respondents were white, almost 40 percent were African American, and less than 5 percent were Latino. Almost 80 percent of the target group had or expected to have Medicaid coverage. Although a smaller 61 percent of the outside group reported similar Medicaid status, this percentage is substantial and indicates that their experiences can be interpreted as those of potential Medicaid recipients.

Table 7
Comparison of Target Population and Other Exit Interview Respondents

Characteristic	Percentage of Group	
	Target Group (N=89)	Outside Group (N=93)
Female	60.7	6.5***
Race/ethnicity		
African American	38.2	39.8
Hispanic/Latino	2.3	5.4
White	59.6	54.8
Have or expect to have Medicaid	78.7*	61.3*
Why approached the Decision Helper+		
Saw it before	15.7	12.9
Told by public assistance specialist	3.4	1.1
Saw the "Nina" poster	32.6	15.1**
Heard about it from a friend	22.5	63.4***
Saw the computer in office	57.3	22.6***
Other reasons	28.1	26.9
Used the Decision Helper today	53.9	85.0***
For users, first time of use	97.9	94.9
For users, situation of use+		
Was alone	33.3	10.1***
Accompanied by children	14.6	0***
Accompanied by adults	56.3	88.6***

* $p < 0.05$ ** $p < 0.01$ *** $p < 0.001$

+ Respondents were allowed to provide one or more of the response options

The target and outside groups also differed in their reasons for approaching the Decision Helper, the percentage who used the Decision Helper, and how they used it. For the target group, the most important reasons for approaching the Decision Helper were that they saw it in the office (57.3 percent), they saw the Nina poster (32.6 percent), or they heard about it from friends (22.5 percent). For the outside user group, the predominant reason they reported was hearing about it from friends (63.4 percent). Some in this group also reported seeing the computer and the Nina poster, but the percentages reporting those reasons were much smaller than for the target group (22.6 and 15.1 percent respectively). An estimated 54 percent of the target group and 85 percent of the outside group used the Decision Helper. These sessions were the first times of use for over 95 percent of both groups. Situations of use also differed for the two groups. Almost 90 percent of the outside group were accompanied by friends when they used the system, whereas only 56 percent of the target group used it with friends.

Use rates of the Decision Helper are shown in Table 8, comparing use by demographic characteristics, Medicaid status, and status in the Economic Service office. Although men were more likely than women to use the Decision Helper, this result is influenced by the outside user group, which was predominantly male. Differences in use rates by race/ethnicity were not significant. With respect to Medicaid status, those who expected to have Medicaid or did not know if they would have it were more likely to use the Decision Helper than those who already were in Medicaid or did not expect to have it. Persons who had completed their appointments with a public assistance specialist (PAS) or did not have an appointment, were more likely to use the Decision Helper than those who were still waiting for their appointments.

Table 8
Use of the Decision Helper by User Characteristics and Medicaid Status

Characteristic	Number With Characteristic	Percentage Who Used Decision Helper [1]
All respondents (N=182)	182	69.8
Gender		
Female	60	48.3***
Male	122	80.3***
Race/ethnicity		
White	104	67.3
Non-white	78	73.1
Medicaid status		
Have Medicaid now	43	60.5*
Expect to have Medicaid	84	77.4*
Do not know if will have Medicaid	13	84.6*
Do not expect to have Medicaid	42	59.5*
Meeting with public assistance specialist		
Already met with PAS	36	88.9**
Waiting to meet with PAS	75	57.3**
Do not have an appointment	71	73.2**
Thought the Decision Helper contained:		
Welfare benefits information	24	62.5*
Medicaid HMO information	144	74.3*
Other	4	50.0*
Do not know	10	30.0*

* p < 0.05   ** p < 0.01   *** p < 0.001

[1] The denominator is all individuals who approached the Decision Helper and looked at it for at least 30 seconds, whether or not they actually went past the first page. Users were those who reported on the exit interview that they had work through at least part of the system.

Use of the Decision Helper was found to be related to people's perceptions of what it contained. The vast majority of persons thought it contained Medicaid HMO information (74.3 percent), and a substantial percentage thought it contained information on welfare benefits (62.5 percent).

Several questions were asked in the exit interviews to examine the extent to which previous experience with Medicaid or with use of computers influenced whether people chose to use the Decision Helper. Because these questions were asked on only one of the two interview forms, responses were obtained for 95 respondents (slightly greater than half the total number of respondents). The results are summarized in Table 9. Fairly small percentages of respondents reported having previous Medicaid experience in either Florida (12.6 percent) or in other states (26.3 percent). Although differences in Decision Helper use rates based on previous Medicaid experience were not statistically significant, individuals who had no previous Medicaid experience were more likely to use the Decision Helper than those with no previous experience.

A fairly high level of computer experience was reported by respondents: 80 percent had used a computer, 73.7 percent had used an ATM, and 95.8 percent had used video games. We found no differences in the percentage who used the Decision Helper based on previous experience with any of these three types of automated systems.

Table 9
Use of the Decision Helper by Amount of Experience with Medicaid and Computers

Characteristic	Number With Characteristic	Percentage Who Used Decision Helper
Subset of respondents	95	74.7
Experience with Medicaid		
Has had Florida Medicaid before	12	66.7
Has not had Florida Medicaid	61	80.3
Missing	22	63.6
Has had other Medicaid before	25	64.0
Has not had other Medicaid	70	78.6
Experience with computers		
Has used a computer	76	75.0
Has never used a computer	10	73.7
Has used an ATM	70	75.7
Has never used an ATM	25	72.0
Has played video games	91	74.7
Has never played a video game	4	75.0

Individuals who did not use the Decision Helper were asked why they did not do so. As shown in Table 10, the predominant responses were that there were too many people using it (41.8 percent) or they had other things to do (18.2 percent). A number of other responses also were given, but the number of persons citing each reason was small. The next most frequent responses--given by three people each--were embarrassment in using the Decision Helper, inability to see well enough to use it, and already knowing the information it provided.

Table 10
Reasons Why Individuals Did Not Use the Decision Helper

Reason	Number (Percentage)
Too many users	23 (41.8)
Had other things to do	10 (18.2)
Embarrassed to use it	3 (5.5)
Cannot see well enough	3 (5.5)
Already know the information	3 (5.5)
The Decision Helper was moved away	2 (3.6)
Decision Helper not working	1 (1.8)
Not able to read	1 (1.8)
Could not hear the sound	1 (1.8)
Other reasons	8 (14.6)

People who used the Decision Helper during the exit interview period were asked additional questions about what they liked and did not like about the system and their assessment of some of the system's features. Table 11 contains frequencies of responses to questions about what the users liked most and least about the Decision Helper, listed in descending order of frequency. Respondents could give more than one answer to these open-ended questions, and frequencies are shown for the first and second responses.

The features people liked most about the Decision Helper was that it is easy and fast to use and it gives a lot of information. Other popular features were Nina's voice, the explanations and definitions provided, the plan comparison ratings, and touch screen navigation. When asked what they liked least about the Decision Helper, the predominant response people gave was the slowness in moving between screens and printing out pages to take home.

In addition to answering open-ended questions about the Decision Helper, users were asked to assess several aspects of the system, including the length of time it took to use the Decision Helper, ease of use, usefulness of the "stars" chart, and use of the printer. As shown in Table 12, 86.6 percent of users thought the Decision Helper was *very* or *somewhat easy* to use, and only 11.8 percent thought it was *too long*. Over 80 percent of users saw the "stars" chart. Of those persons who saw the "stars" chart, 93.1 percent thought it was *very or somewhat easy* to use and 94.1 percent said the information was helpful in making health plan choices. The printer was used by 44.1 percent of users to print Decision Helper information. Another 16.5 percent reported they could not use the printer because it was out of paper.

Table 11
Reactions of Users to the Decision Helper

Decision Helper Feature	Number (Percentage) Who Identified the Feature*	
	First Response	Second Response
What liked most about the Decision Helper		
Easy and fast to use	28 (22.1)	2 (1.6)
Gives a lot of information	24 (18.9)	8 (6.3)
Nina's voice	16 (12.6)	8 (6.3)
Explanations and definitions	14 (11.2)	5 (3.9)
The plan comparison ratings	10 (7.9)	3 (2.4)
Touch screen navigation	9 (7.1)	3 (2.4)
Information on Medicaid	6 (4.7)	2 (1.6)
Information on benefits	4 (3.2)	3 (2.4)
Graphics and pictures	3 (2.4)	3 (2.4)
List of doctors	3 (2.4)	3 (2.4)
Availability, access of the system	3 (2.4)	
Print information to take home	2 (1.6)	2 (1.6)
Information on how to choose a plan	2 (1.6)	4 (3.2)
Other	1 (0.8)	1 (0.8)
No response	2 (1.6)	80 (63.0)
What liked least about the Decision Helper		
Too slow between screens, printing	29 (22.8)	1 (0.8)
Confusing, hard to understand	6 (4.7)	1 (0.8)
Not loud enough	6 (4.7)	1 (0.8)
Too crowded around computer	6 (4.7)	
Small buttons hard to touch right	4 (3.2)	
Do not like touching screen, machines	4 (3.2)	
Do not like standing to use it	3 (2.4)	
Do not agree with ratings	2 (1.6)	
Too much on one screen	2 (1.6)	
Other **	8 (6.3)	2 (1.6)
Reported there were no problems	5 (3.9)	
No response	52 (40.9)	122 (96.1)

* Respondents may offer one or more responses to these open-ended questions. The first and second responses are reported here.

** Other responses included: does not have needed information, Nina was not real, music was too loud, bad location, computer was too fast, needed better voice for Nina, and program was not interactive.

Table 12
Assessment of the Decision Helper by Users

Decision Helper Feature	Percentage
Ease of use	
Very easy	56.7
Somewhat easy	29.9
Somewhat hard	8.7
Very hard	3.2
The Decision Helper was too long	11.8
Saw screen with "stars" chart	81.1
Ease of understanding the "stars" chart+	
Very easy	57.2
Somewhat easy	35.9
Somewhat hard	5.8
Very hard	1.0
Stars information helps plan choice+	94.2
Use of printer	
Printed DH information	44.1
Did not use printer	39.4
Printer out of paper	16.5

+   Percentage of individuals who reported they saw the screen with the stars chart (N=103).

Interviews with Staff Involved with the Field Test

Approximately six weeks after the end of the Decision Helper field test, the RAND team performed a site visit to conduct interviews with governmental personnel and others who were actively involved in operating the Daytona Beach field test. As discussed in Section 3, these individuals included the two staff persons at the local Economic Services Office who worked with us on the field test and the computer systems expert with whom RAND contracted to provide technical support for computer repairs and data transfers during the field test. In addition, during interviews with AHCA and Medicaid staff in Tallahassee, we asked for their reactions to the Decision Helper and suggestions for improvements. Although general support was expressed for the Decision Helper as an informational vehicle, some issues also were identified that must be addressed for such a system to be implemented successfully. The following were the strengths and weaknesses identified about the system during the interviews.

Strengths of the Decision Helper:

- The physician directory, which allowed users to look up the plans in which their physician participates, was an important feature. Consumers consistently say that information about their doctors is one of the items that they most want to know, and our field test provided further evidence of this priority.
- The animated host (Nina) was engaging. However, she could be made more effective by adding more movement, including more features to help with navigation, such as pointing to buttons.

- The print capability was important. Users wanted to take home the list of plans for their doctor and the comparison screens.
- The audio capability was very helpful in engaging users and reducing the amount of reading they must do. The audio could be refined to depart even further from the text.
- Although opinions were somewhat mixed, the majority of interviewees favored the linear design of the program's navigation, for simplicity's sake, over a menu-driven system. The linear design would have been even more satisfactory if the physician directory (which was of most interest to users) came first and if users could receive printouts at any point in the session, for greater flexibility in terminating their use of the system after their information needs are met.
- The presence of the Decision Helper in the Economic Services Office imposed little burden on the staff of the Office. The person responsible for keeping the machine in operation usually checked it about once an hour and as little as 2-3 times a day when she was busy with other things. The biggest issue was security, which required the additional task of rolling the cart in and out of the waiting room each day.
- Having an outside technical person was essential. Support for information systems within the Economic Services Office was stretched very thin and was not necessarily on location and on call, even for the office's own internal emergencies. The Economic Services Office would not have undertaken the project if it had been expected to provide its own technical support.

Weaknesses of the Decision Helper:

- The location of the computer in the waiting room of the Economic Services Office discouraged use of the system. The room was noisy, and there were many children running around. There was no privacy; so anyone using the system was observed by others sitting in the waiting room, which could be intimidating.
- People did not necessarily know that they were going to qualify for Medicaid (and would need to choose a Medicaid health plan) when they were sitting in the waiting room. The Decision Helper would be more relevant to people after they completed their eligibility interview with a case worker and were on their way out of the office.
- On the other hand, potential users often are young parents accompanied by their children. Typically, they are in a hurry to get their children out of the Economic Services Offices as quickly as possible. To encourage these mothers to stop and use the Decision Helper thoughtfully, some kind of entertainment for their children would need to be provided.
- Given the above observations, virtually everyone interviewed thought that the system would have been more effective if, at the conclusion of the eligibility interview, caseworkers had referred likely Medicaid eligibles to a semi-private location where they could use the Decision Helper.
- The system did not inform users that print commands had registered, so users pressed the print button repeatedly, with resulting prints of many copies of the same page.
- More voice instructions and other navigational help are needed (see discussion of Nina above).
- The program is too slow. Screen changes, searches, and printing should be quicker.

- An adjustable volume control should be available to the user. Sometimes the room sound level is high and must be overcome by users. At other times the Decision Helper is too loud, interfering with others in the room and compromising the users' privacy.
- Some interviewees thought Nina's dress and appearance were too provocative. The impression of feminine "frilliness" may have been reinforced by her name, since Nina means "little girl" in Spanish.

Section 6

ISSUES AND POLICY IMPLICATIONS

Although the paper report and Decision Helper are quite distinct formats for presenting health plan performance information, the Florida Medicaid demonstration revealed a number of issues involved in communicating information effectively to users that were common to both media. In this discussion, we consider the insights this demonstration has offered us, with particular focus on the research questions we posed in Section 1. We first address some overall conclusions we have reached on factors for successful implementation and adaptability of the CAHPS report templates for a Medicaid population. Then we examine lessons from field testing each of the paper report and Decision Helper.

OVERALL IMPLEMENTATION ISSUES

Our first research question sought information on which conditions were necessary or important to achieve success in implementing CAHPS reports for a Medicaid population. In this demonstration, we identified four general dimensions of a consumer information strategy:

- The types, amounts, and display of the plan performance information itself;
- The design of the report medium, including the paper report document and the software and hardware of the Decision Helper;
- The physical environment in which the information is provided to potential users; and
- The timing of information availability relative to when plan choices are being made.

A clear high-level finding was that failures in any of these dimensions can impede the communication process if the failures lead to consumers' not noticing the reports or discourage them from spending time with the information. Recognizing the virtual impossibility of achieving a "perfect" implementation capability, our analysis of demonstration results focused on identifying the elements that appeared to be most important for successful dissemination of comparative health plan information to Medicaid beneficiaries. Because these differed somewhat for the paper reports and Decision Helper, this issue is considered in more detail in our discussion of each of these report formats.

With respect to our research question regarding the ability to adapt the CAHPS formats for use with a Medicaid population, substantial changes had to be made in both the paper report template and the Decision Helper to make them more accessible to the user. We believe, however, that this simplification process may be appropriate for any users of the reports, given strong feedback that people will be discouraged from using the reports if they are difficult to work with or understand. Our field experience in Florida also reinforces the importance of soliciting feedback from users during the design of plan performance reports. Surprising details were found to influence users' receptivity to the reports.

Both the focus groups that examined the paper report and the exit interviews from the Decision Helper field test revealed that Florida Medicaid beneficiaries were interested in the comparative health plan information. Most of those interviewed reported that they found the information to be useful and easy to interpret, although some were confused about interpretation of the stars. At the same time, participants expressed a diversity of opinions regarding the report contents, format, and timing of presentation.

This feedback from beneficiaries highlights the importance of continuing to build an evidence-based foundation that defines the basic elements required to communicate plan performance information effectively, while allowing flexibility to tailor specific report design and dissemination to the preferences of each sponsor and the populations it serves. Whereas we understand there is no one "correct answer" for report design, empirical knowledge has not yet clearly identified what are the essential and discretionary elements of presentation.

ASSESSMENT OF THE PAPER REPORT

We found differing information for the paper report and Decision Helper with respect to our research question on the receptivity of Medicaid consumers to plan performance reports. For the paper report, Medicaid recipients gave us mixed feedback on the plan performance information itself as well as the way it was presented.

An underlying issue in the focus group feedback about the paper report involved the extent to which they trusted the survey information. This issue took two forms — concerns that the survey sample did not necessarily represent them as individuals, and concerns about the objectivity of the survey itself. Some of the participants who challenged the representativeness of the sample appeared to not fully understand the concept of random samples. Others challenged the sample because it indeed was a mix of people who, on average, might have health plan or service needs that differed from an individual's specific needs. Symptomatic of this issue was the request by several participants for survey information for narrowly defined population groups (e.g., by the nature of Medicaid eligibility or those with children with chronic health conditions). Most questions regarding the objectivity of the survey appeared to be motivated by suspicions that health plans may have influenced the survey results. We have found similar responses in other CAHPS evaluation work, including laboratory experiments and our demonstration with the New Jersey Medicaid program (Spranca et al., in press; Farley et al., submitted).

Our focus group results suggest that the placement of the survey information at the back of the *Here Are Your Choices* booklet contributed to the trust issues. Some questions might be alleviated by placing the survey information at the front of the booklet, so users could see it before they actually reviewed the plan performance results. However, because budget constraints preclude generating detailed survey information for many specific sub-groups, issues regarding the representativeness of the sample are likely to remain. This issue points toward the future value of computerized reports, as well as to the value of providing some decision support methods that help users to focus on performance dimensions that are important to them and to apply the group results to their own circumstances.

With respect to our research question about what features of the report are important, feedback from focus group participants highlighted their desire for the report to contain information on the plan features and covered benefits, as well as the comparative performance information. Although we preferred consolidation of all this information into one report, it was not possible to make such large-scale changes to the Florida Medicaid documents for the sake of this demonstration. We believe that such a comprehensive presentation can help strengthen the plan choice process by giving beneficiaries easy access to the full set of information they should be considering.

Focus group participants also expressed a preference for a visually attractive report that was easy to read. The options for report layout were severely constrained by the Medicaid program's existing production and mailing requirements. The size of the mailing envelope and AHCA's very limited printing budget contributed to producing a visually uninteresting document that was not easy to use because the placement of the staple made it difficult to read the backs of pages. Although these factors may be relatively fixed in the short term, a Medicaid program is able to make substantial changes in its information materials over a longer-term period. A more difficult issue is whether to produce one state-wide report or a set of separate reports for individual counties or cluster of counties served by the same health plans. The separate county reports likely would be more useful to beneficiaries, but they also would entail much larger production, mailing, and administrative costs for the Medicaid program.

ASSESSMENT OF THE DECISION HELPER

We learned quickly that our research question regarding the optimal circumstances for providing a computer-based system addressed the key issue for successful use of the Decision Helper. Although RAND's initial attention during the demonstration was on the design of the Decision Helper software and related computer hardware, our span of view quickly expanded to also consider workspace and environmental conditions as we prepared to go into the field in the Daytona Beach Economic Services Office. Throughout this process, the design guidance given by state and local staff who worked with the Medicaid beneficiaries proved to be generally on target. For the software product itself, we created a simple linear navigational path, limited the amount of text, provided an animated host that talked to the user, and installed touch screen capability. We also programmed print capability into the system, which was reported by users to be an important feature. As we prepared to set up the system in the Daytona Beach office, the environmental conditions became a design focus, including establishing an acceptable workspace configuration and providing security protections.

The field test documented low use rates for the Decision Helper. Computer logs recorded an average of 25 sessions per day during the first two weeks of the demonstration period, most of which did not get past the first screen. Similar results were obtained from our two-day observation period, where we estimated that 8.4 percent of those entering the Economic Services Office approached the computer and only half of them used it for more than one minute. We had anticipated that only a fraction of potential users would find this medium attractive. Indeed, some individuals reported in the exit interviews that they simply were not interested in the Decision Helper. However, use rates were lower than expected.

With respect to our research question on the computer literacy of Medicaid recipients, this issue did not appear to be a constraint for use of the Decision Helper. Exit interview respondents reported high use rates of computer-based systems. Close to 88 percent of them had used a computer, 74 percent had used an ATM, and 96 percent had played video games.

In this context, we turned our attention to identifying other barriers that might be limiting their use of the system. Not surprisingly, possible deterrents to use of the Decision Helper cut across the four basic information strategy dimensions. Two important factors identified were the timing for access to the Decision Helper and the environmental issue of privacy. Although the Economic Services Office was the best location we could identify to gain access to the Medicaid population, it was not ideal. Individuals tend to be thinking more about their welfare benefits — not Medicaid benefits — when they are in this office. The exit interviews provided indirect evidence that this timing issue may be important, in that people who approached the Decision Helper after they had completed their case worker interviews were more likely to use it, compared with those who were still waiting for their appointments. The focus groups raised a counter-argument, however, where some participants reported they wanted the information early in their Medicaid enrollment process.

With respect to the issue of privacy, a few individuals participating in the exit interviews indicated they were embarrassed to use the Decision Helper. We infer from these responses that the source of embarrassment was the location of the system in the office waiting area where everyone in the area could observe what Decision Helper users were doing. This feedback may be an indicator that larger numbers of individuals were discouraged from using the system. Recognizing that the conduct of the exit interviews artificially increased use of the Decision Helper, this privacy issue may be even larger than what we observed.

For the research question regarding which features were important to Medicaid consumers, we obtained information from users that highlighted the uniqueness of a Decision Helper application. In general, this feedback reinforced the principle that "simpler is better" for both the contents of the information provided and navigational aspects of the system. Users responded positively to the touch screen feature and the ability to print out pages to take home. Problems they experienced using the system highlighted the need to provide simple instructions on the first screen for how to use the system, to ensure system speed to move quickly through the screens, and to show a dialogue box confirming that a print request was being executed.

We were reminded that the layout of each screen needs to conform to the reality that the English language reads from the top left to the bottom right of a page. The first item that users saw on the Decision Helper screen was the check box that showed them where they were in the 4 sections of the system. Many individuals were observed trying to use that box as a menu to move to the section they wanted to see when, in fact, the navigational buttons were placed on the bottom center of the screen. In addition to the navigational issue raised, this behavior might also be a sign that users would appreciate a simple menu that enabled them to move directly to plan ratings or to doctor affiliations. It may not be necessary to retain the full simplicity of the linear path designed for the Florida Medicaid Decision Helper.

Other aspects of the Decision Helper product itself that we found needed careful management were the robustness of the system software and hardware to operate for extended periods of time and the daily maintenance requirements for the local office staff. Equipment security issues with respect to damage and theft were both more important and more complex than we had believed at the start of the field test. In fact, we had to make some tradeoffs between goals for security and ease of use when selecting the console case and mounting the computer and printer in the case. The demonstration also substantiated the need to have external technical expertise available to troubleshoot problems. However, because the Decision Helper was in daily operation for only 2 weeks before the on-site evaluation began, this placement did not fully test the viability of the system under long-term operating conditions.

DISCUSSION

The demonstration in Florida showed that multiple design and implementation factors can affect the success of efforts to report CAHPS survey findings to consumers. Although this finding applies equally to the paper report and Decision Helper, our experience with placing the Florida Medicaid Decision Helper in the field highlights the importance of managing complex factors to give beneficiaries the best ease of access to comparative plan information.

This lesson also has important implications for CAHPS evaluations (Carman et al., 1999). First, it means that one should not be quick to generalize from the success or failure of any particular implementation of CAHPS (or "consumer report cards" more generally). A slightly different implementation might have very different results. Second, each sponsor that uses CAHPS needs to exercise considerable care and flexibility to make sure that their implementation is fine-tuned to the specifics of their particular situation.

The Florida experience points to the importance of including other information, along with the CAHPS survey findings, in reports that are given to consumers. Beneficiaries in the focus groups identified a broad range of information they also want to have, most of which was available in a separate report but not presented together with the plan performance information. In addition, the information on plan affiliations of physicians was one of the most popular features of the Decision Helper.

The collective findings of the Florida Medicaid demonstration offer persuasive support for the premise that CAHPS and other plan performance information can provide value for Medicaid beneficiaries. Participants interpreted the stars effectively to make plan comparisons, and they tended to approach the task with a healthy skepticism that yielded realistic interpretations of the information before them. What effects this information may have on their actual health plan choices, however, remain to be tested before any conclusions can be drawn regarding the effects of CAHPS. Given the large size of the Medicaid populations across the states, Medicaid CAHPS could contribute substantially to helping large numbers of beneficiaries make more informed plan choices — if they choose to use the information.

REFERENCES

Baron, Jonathan, *Thinking and Deciding*, Cambridge University Press, New York, NY, 1988.

Carman K. L., P. F. Short, D. O. Farley, J. A. Schnaier, D. B. Elliott, P. M. Gallagher, "Epilogue: Early lessons from CAHPS™ Demonstrations and Evaluations," *Medical Care*, 37(3):MS97-105, 1999.

Castles, A, P. Goodwin, Cheryl Damberg, Consumer Use of Quality of Care Information: An Evalaution of California Consumer HealthScope (abstract), *Abstract Book of the Association of Health Service Research* 14:171-2, 1997.

Chernew, Michael, and Dennis P. Scanlon, Health Plan Report Cards and Insurance Choice, *Inquiry* 35(1):9-22, Spring 1998.

Crofton, Christine, James Lubalin, and Charles Darby, Foreword, Supplement, *Medical Care* 37(3):MS1-MS9, March 1999.

Davis, Karen, Karen Scott Collins, Cathy Schoen, and Cynthia Morris, Choice Matters: Enrollees' Views of their Health Plans, *Health Affairs* 14(2):99-112, Summer 1995.

Farley, D. O., Pamela F. Short, Marc Elliott, et al., "Effects of CAHPS Health Care Plan Performance Information on Plan Choices by New Jersey Medicaid Beneficiaries," submitted, 2000.

Gibbs, Deborah A, Judith A. Sangl, and Barri Burrus, Consumer Perspectives on Information Needs for Health Plan Choice, *Health Care Financing Review* 18(1):31-54, Fall 1996.

Health Care Financing Administration, Medicaid Managed Care State Enrollment – June 1998, published on web site (www.hcfa.gov/medicaid/plansum8.htm).

Hibbard, JH, JJ Jewett. Will Quality Report Cards Help Consumers? *Health Affairs* 16(3):218-228, May-June 1997.

Hibbard, JH, P Slovic, JJ Jewett. Informing Consumer Decisions in Health Care: Implications from Decision-Making Research, *Milbank Quarterly* 75(3):395-414, 1997.

Hibbard, JH, S Sofaer, JJ Jewett. Condition-Specific Performance Information: Assessing Salience, Comprehension, and Approaches for Communicating Quality, *Health Care Financing Review* 18(1):95-109, Fall 1996.

Knutson, DJ, N Dahms, E Kind, Jeanne McGee, M Finch, JB Fowles, The Effect of Health Plan Report Cards on Consumer Knowledge, Attitudes and Plan Choice: A Quasi-Experimental Evaluation (abstract), Abstract Book of the Association of Health Service Research 14:184, 1997.

Marquis, M. Susan, and Jeannette A. Rogowski, *Participation in Alternative Health Plans*, RAND/R-4105-HCFA, RAND, Santa Monica, CA, 1991.

Mechanic, David, Therese Ettel, Diane Davis, Choosing Among Health Insurance Options: A Study of New Employees, *Inquiry* 27:14-23, Spring 1990.

McGee, Jeanne, David E. Kanouse, Shoshanna Sofaer, J. Lee Hargraves, Elizabeth Hot, Susan Kleiman. Making Survey Results Easy to Report to Consumers: How Reporting Needs Guided Survey Design in CAHPS, *Medical Care*, 37(3):MS32-MS40, 1999.

Payne, John W., James R. Bettman, Eric J. Johnson, *The Adaptive Decision Maker*, Cambridge University Press, New York, NY, 1993.

Robinson, Sandra, and Mollyann Brodie, Understanding the Quality Challenge for Health Consumers: The Kaiser/AHCPR Survey, *Joint Commission Journal on Quality Improvement* 23(5):239-44, May 1997.

Sainfort, Francois, and Bridge C. Booske, Role of Information in Consumer Selection of Health Plans, *Health Care Financing Review* 18(1):31-54, Fall 1996.

Scanlon, Dennis P., Michael Chernew, Judith R. Lave, Consumer Health Plan Choice: Current Knowledge and Future Directions, *Annual Review of Public Health* 18:507-28, 1997.

Spranca, Mark E., David E. Kanouse, Pamela Farley Short, Donna O. Farley, Ron D. Hays, Do Consumer Reports of Health Plan Quality Affect Health Plan Selection? *Health Services Research*, in press.

Tumlinson, A., A. Hendricks, EM Stone, P Mahoney, and H. Bottigheimer, Choosing a Health Plan: What Information will Consumers Use? *Health Affairs* 16(3):229-38, May-June 1997.

Appendix A
PERFORMANCE DIMENSIONS FOR FLORIDA MEDICAID PLANS

GLOBAL RATINGS

Overall, how would you rate your Medicaid health plan.

How would you rate your regular doctor (or nurse) overall.

PERFORMANCE COMPOSITES (time reference – last 6 months)

Choosing the health plan again

Given what you now know about your Medicaid health plan, would you choose it as your health plan again.

Getting the care they need

How many times did you get medical care at a doctor's office, clinic, or hospital emergency room.

Were you always able to see a specialist when you needed to.

Getting care without long waits

How long have you usually had to wait between the time you made an appointment and the day you saw a doctor for: a minor illness or injury; urgent care

Was there ever a time when you were unable to get an appointment with a doctor (or nurse) as soon as you wanted.

Once you arrived for a scheduled appointment, how long did you usually have to wait to see a doctor (or nurse)

Doctors or nurses communicating well with patients

Has a doctor (or nurse) every failed to treat you with courtesy and respect.

Have you ever felt that a doctor (or nurse) failed to listen carefully to you.

Has a doctor (or nurse) ever failed to explain things to you in a way you could understand.

Doctors or nurses spending enough time and knowing medical history

Has a doctor (or nurse) ever spent less time with you than you thought was needed.

Did you ever see a doctor (or nurse) who seemed to know too little about your medical history.

Doctors or nurses talking with patients about preventing health problems

Has your regular doctor (or nurse) every talked with you about diet or exercise.

Has your regular doctor (or nurse) every talked with you about smoking or use of tobacco.

Has your regular doctor (or nurse) every talked with you or reminded you about getting preventive care such as routine physicals, shots, or mammograms.

Whether they complained to their plan

Have you called or written your Medicaid health plan about a complaint or problem.

Having good doctors or nurses to choose from

How would you rate your Medicaid health plan on the number of doctors and other health care providers you can choose from.

How would you rate your Medicaid health plan on the quality of the doctors and other health care providers you can choose from.

Appendix B

FLORIDA MEDICAID BOOKLET

HERE ARE YOUR CHOICES-MEDICAID HEALTH PLANS IN VOLUSIA COUNTY, FLORIDA

Here Are Your Choices

Medicaid Health Plans in Volusia County

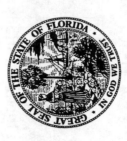

Agency for Health Care Administration

If you receive Medicaid, then you have to choose a Medicaid health plan.

However, there are some exceptions. If any of the following are true, then you do not need to choose a Medicaid health plan:

☑ you are in the Medically Needy program

☑ you live in a nursing home, hospice, or other facility

☑ you are receiving temporary Medicaid benefits while you are pregnant

☑ you are eligible for both Medicaid and Medicare

How will this booklet help you choose a Medicaid health plan?

It is important for you to choose your health plan. If you don't choose one, then one will be chosen for you.

This booklet has a new kind of information to help you choose the best plan for you and your family.

This booklet shows what people thought about the Medicaid health plan (HMO or MediPass) they were in. It will help you choose the best health plan for you and your family.

This booklet gives information about the two HMOs and MediPass in your county.

Where did this information come from?

People were given a survey that asked them questions about their Medicaid health plans (HMO or MediPass). They rated their plans and told about the care they received, their doctors (or nurses), and their health plan. Page 10 has more information about this survey.

What do the stars mean?

The stars are used to represent survey results. They show what people thought about the care they received, their doctors (or nurses), and their health plan.

★★★ = This plan did better than other plans in your county.

★★ = This plan did average for plans in your county.

★ = This plan did less well than other plans in your county.

What are HMOs and MediPass?

When you choose your Medicaid health plan, you must decide to join either an HMO or MediPass.

This page tells you how HMOs and MediPass are the same and how they are different.

You can choose from three health plans in your county. One plan is MediPass. The other two plans are Health Maintenance Organizations (HMOs).

How are HMOs and MediPass the same?

☑ You choose a regular doctor (or nurse) who will keep track of your health care. This person is your primary care provider.

☑ You choose your regular doctor (or nurse) from a list that is given to you by the HMO or by MediPass.

☑ Your regular doctor (or nurse) will send you to see a specialist or to the hospital if you need one.

☑ You can always call your regular doctor (or nurse) if you need

- a check-up
- specialist care
- shots
- medical supplies or equipment
- advice about a health problem

How are HMOs and MediPass different?

☑ With an HMO, you get your care through its network of hospitals, doctors, nurses, and other health care providers. Your regular doctor (or nurse) may refer you to any specialist who is in the HMO's network.

☑ With MediPass, you have more doctors and nurses to choose from. Your regular doctor (or nurse) may refer you to any specialist who accepts Medicaid patients.

☑ In addition to the basic package of health care services, HMOs offer extra benefits such as programs on quitting smoking, substance abuse, domestic violence, pregnancy prevention, pregnancy, and children's wellness.

How do you use this booklet to choose an HMO or MediPass?

Remember that the plan you choose can make a big difference in the quality of care you get.

This booklet will help you make an informed choice about the plan that is best for you and your family.

Look at the steps on the right to find out how to use this booklet.

Step 1

Go to page 4 to see what people thought, overall, about:

- their health plans and
- their regular doctor (or nurse).

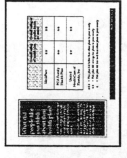

Step 2

Go to page 5 to learn more about the things that the survey asked people about. As you read, think about which of these things are important to you.

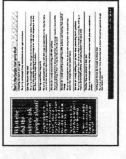

Step 3

Go to pages 6–8 to see what people like you thought about the plans they were in. In the upper left hand corner, check either "Yes" or "No" to remind yourself if you think this plan did well on the things that are important to you.

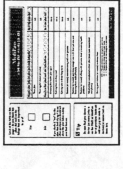

Step 4

Go to page 9 to:

- list the plans that you checked "Yes" for on pages 6–8, and
- learn about other important questions you should ask about plans before you make a final decision.

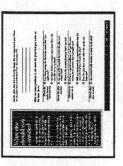

What did people like you think about their health plan?

Look at the chart on the right to see what people thought, overall, of their health plans and their regular doctor (or nurse).

The survey also asked people about eight other things. The next page has definitions of these things. Pages 6–8 show you how each plan in your county did on these things.

	Overall rating of health plan	Overall rating of regular doctor (or nurse)
MediPass	★★	★★
PCA Family Health Plan	★★	★★
United HealthCare of Florida, Inc.	★★	★★

★★★ = This plan did better than other plans in your county.

★★ = This plan did average for plans in your county.

★ = This plan did less well than other plans in your county.

What else did the survey ask people about?

The eight things that the survey asked about are listed on the right. You may think that some of these are important. You may not care about others. Read about them and decide which are important to you.

Pages 6–8 show you how people thought their plan did on each of these things.

It's best to choose a health plan that does well on the things that you think are important.

Here's what people were asked about

Choosing the health plan again

The survey asked people if they would choose the plan again in the future.

Getting the care they need

The survey asked people how often they got the care they thought they needed. This includes getting to see a specialist, getting care in the evenings or on weekends, and getting to see their own doctor (or nurse) when they thought they needed to.

Getting care without long waits

The survey asked people how long it took them to get an appointment or how long they had to wait to see their doctor (or nurse) once they arrived for a scheduled appointment.

Doctors (or nurses) communicating well with patients

The survey asked people if their doctors (or nurses) treated them with courtesy, listened to them carefully, and explained things to them in a way that they could understand.

Doctors (or nurses) spending enough time with patients and knowing their medical history

The survey asked people how often their doctors (or nurses) spent enough time with them and if their doctors (or nurses) knew enough about their medical history.

Doctors (or nurses) talking with patients about preventing health problems

The survey asked people how often their regular doctor (or nurse) talked to them about exercise, diet, smoking, or ways to prevent health problems, such as getting physical check-ups or shots.

Whether they complained to their plan

MediPass

1–800–940–4803 OR 1–904–238–4803

People were asked to give an overall rating for	How the plan did
Their plan	★★
Their regular doctor (or nurse)	★★

People in this plan were also asked about	How the plan did
Choosing the health plan again	★★★
Getting the care they need	★★★
Getting care without long waits	★★★
Doctors (or nurses) communicating well with patients	★★
Doctors (or nurses) spending enough time with their patients and knowing their medical history	★★
Doctors (or nurses) talking with patients about preventing health problems	★★
Whether they complained to their plan (more stars means fewer complaints)	★★★
Having good doctors (or nurses) to choose from	★★

★★★ = This plan did better than other plans in your county.
★★ = This plan did average for plans in your county.
★ = This plan did less well than other plans in your county.

Look at the table on this page—do you think this plan did well on the things that are important to you?

☐ *Yes*

☐ *No*

If you checked "Yes" for this plan, then look at page 9 to see other questions you should ask about this plan before making

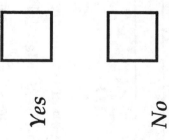 **Tip**

Be sure that you choose a doctor (or nurse) who is on the HMO or MediPass list of providers. Medicaid will not pay for visits to doctors (or nurses) not on these lists.

PCA Family Health Plan

1-800-328-5804

People were asked to give an overall rating for	How the plan did
Their plan	★★
Their regular doctor (or nurse)	★★

People in this plan were also asked about	How the plan did
Choosing the health plan again	★★
Getting the care they need	★★
Getting care without long waits	★
Doctors (or nurses) communicating well with patients	★★
Doctors (or nurses) spending enough time with their patients and knowing their medical history	★★
Doctors (or nurses) talking with patients about preventing health problems	★★
Whether they complained to their plan (more stars means fewer complaints)	★★
Having good doctors (or nurses) to choose from	★★

★★★ = This plan did better than other plans in your county.
★★ = This plan did average for plans in your county.
★ = This plan did less well than other plans in your county.

Look at the table on this page—do you think this plan did well on the things that are important to you?

Yes [ ]

No [ ]

If you checked "Yes" for this plan, then look at page 9 to see other questions you should ask about this plan before making

---

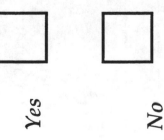

☑ Tip

If you are currently in Children's Medical Services (CMS), you can choose an HMO only if you want to leave CMS. If you want to stay in CMS, you must choose MediPass.

United HealthCare of Florida, Inc.

1-800-899-6550

	How the plan did
People were asked to give an overall rating for	
Their plan	★★
Their regular doctor (or nurse)	★★
People in this plan were also asked about	**How the plan did**
Choosing the health plan again	★★
Getting the care they need	★
Getting care without long waits	★★
Doctors (or nurses) communicating well with patients	★
Doctors (or nurses) spending enough time with their patients and knowing their medical history	★
Doctors (or nurses) talking with patients about preventing health problems	★★
Whether they complained to their plan (more stars means fewer complaints)	★
Having good doctors (or nurses) to choose from	★★

★★★ = This plan did better than other plans in your county.

★★ = This plan did average for plans in your county.

★ = This plan did less well than other plans in your county.

Look at the table on this page—do you think this plan did well on the things that are important to you?

Yes ☐

No ☐

If you checked "Yes" for this plan, then look at page 9 to see other questions you should ask about this plan before making

☑ Tip

For each eligible member of your family, you can choose a different regular doctor (or nurse) from the HMO or MediPass list of providers.

List the plans that did well on the things that are important to you. These are the plans that you checked "Yes" for on pages 6–8.

Here are some questions to ask about the plans that did well.

About the plan's doctors (and nurses)

☐ Can I keep seeing the doctor (or nurse) that I see right now?

☐ Are there doctors (or nurses) near where I live who can take me as a patient?

About the plan services

☐ Are any of the hospitals listed for this plan near where I live?

☐ Where is the nearest pharmacy that I can use?

About your special needs

☐ If I have a special condition, can I get the same treatment or services that I get right now?

☐ Will my treatments for a special condition stop for any period of time if I join the plan?

☐ Does the plan have a provider who speaks my language?

About other plan benefits

☐ Are mental health services covered by the plan?

☐ Are there other services covered by the plan?

What else should you consider?

You have narrowed down your choices by checking "Yes" for the plans that did well on the things that are important to you.

Now, you can narrow the plans more by asking other important questions that are listed on this page.

Before making a final choice, be sure to get more information about the plan's doctors (and nurses), plan services, your special needs, and other plan benefits. You can do this by calling plans, by calling the Choice Counseling hotline, 1-888-367-6554, or by reading the agency's booklet called "The Choice is Yours."

How was the survey done?

Look to the right to find out more about how the survey was done.

- The survey was sponsored by the Florida Agency for Health Care Administration and carried out by Westat, Inc., in the fall of 1996.

- A total of 989 members of 3 health plans across the state of Florida completed a survey. These people had been with their current health plan for at least six months and were chosen to represent all members.

- When the survey was about a child's experiences, answers were given by a parent or other adult.

- The survey was done by mail. Participation was voluntary and confidential.

- Of the plan members who were selected to be in the survey sample, 38 percent mailed back a completed questionnaire.

- Westat and RAND analyzed the survey results, and the American Institutes for Research designed the report with assistance from RAND. The federal Agency for Health Care Policy and Research (AHCPR) funded these efforts.

Appendix C

PROTOCOL MATERIALS FOR FOCUS GROUPS WITH NEW ENROLLEES
FLORIDA MEDICAID DEMONSTRATION

QUESTIONS ABOUT YOU

It would help us to know a little bit about you and to describe the participants in the group discussion. Please take a moment to answer these questions. Since your name is not written on this form no one will know what information you give us. We will not share your individual answers to these items with anyone from Florida Medicaid.

1. How many children under age 18 do you have? (If none, enter 0)

    ____   children

2. What is the highest level of school you have completed?

(Check One Answer)

    ____   8th grade or less
    ____   Some high school or less
    ____   High school diploma or GED
    ____   Vocational school or some college
    ____   College degree
    ____   Professional or graduate degree

3. Are you currently married?

(Check One Answer)

    ____   Yes
    ____   No

4. How do you describe yourself?

(Check One Answer)

    ____   African American or Black
    ____   Hispanic or Latino
    ____   Native American or American Indian
    ____   Asian or Pacific Islander
    ____   White
    ____   Something else (please specify: _____)

5. Our records show that either you or your child were signed up for Medicaid in November or December of 1997. Is this correct? *(Check One Answer)*

    ____   Yes
    ____   No

6.   Who was signed up for Medicaid in November or December of 1997?

(Check All That Apply)

    ____   You
    ____   Your child or children
    ____   Other members of your family

7. Were you (or your child) assigned to a Medicaid health plan by the state, or did you choose a plan?

(Check One Answer)

    ____   Assigned by state
    ____   Chose a plan

8.   What Medicaid plan do you (or your child) belong to?

(Check One Answer)

    ____   MediPass
    ____   PCA Family Health Plan
    ____   United HealthCare of Florida, Inc.
    ____   Some other plan (what is it called?_____)

9.   When you received your Medicaid information packet, did you get a booklet called "Here Are Your Choices - Medicaid Health Plans in Volusia County"?

(Check One Answer)

    ____   Yes
    ____   No ==> PLEASE STOP, THANK YOU FOR COMPLETING THIS FORM
    ____   Don't remember ==> PLEASE STOP, THANK YOU FOR COMPLETING THIS FORM

10.   Did you use the booklet called "Here Are Your Choices - Medicaid Health Plans in Volusia County" to pick your (or your child's) Medicaid health plan?

(Check One Answer)

    ____   Yes
    ____   No

THANK YOU FOR YOUR HELP. PLEASE PUT THIS FORM IN THE ATTACHED ENVELOPE AND SEAL IT.

CAHPS EVALUATION FOCUS GROUPS
DRAFT DISCUSSION GUIDE

I. Introduction (est. 5 minutes)
    A. Explain the general purpose and format of the focus group.
        Purpose: Get your feedback on materials that other people on Medicaid will use to choose a health plan.
    B.   Reassure participants about confidentiality. Remind them to use first names only. Explain purpose of audio taping.
    C. Introduce observers (if any) and ask participants to introduce themselves.
        Ice breaker: What do you like about living in Florida?

II. Warm-Up Exercise (est. 10 minutes)
    A. Ask participants to complete questionnaire about themselves (a.k.a. demographic items). Questionnaire will be distributed with an envelope. Participants will place questionnaire in envelope and seal it.
    Purpose: I'd like you to give us some information about you that I can use to describe participants in today's group. I don't want you to write your name on it and your individual forms will not be shared with anyone from the state of Florida. Completing the form is voluntary whether you complete it or not will not effect any benefits you may receive.

III. Florida Report "Here Are Your Choices" (est. 50-60 minutes)
    A. HAND OUT REPORTS. This booklet contains information about the health plans available to people in Volusia county who are on Medicaid. It is sent out along with the general information packet about Medicaid.
    PROBE: Who here has received a booklet like this from the county? (When?)

Let's turn to page 1 of the booklet (How will this booklet help you).
    Take a moment to look this page over. (allow a few moments for participants to read the page).
    PROBE: What do you notice most on this page? (Do you think that is useful to know?) What else do you notice? Is the information on this page helpful?
    PROBE: Would you trust the information in this booklet? Where do you think the information came from?

Let's turn the page . . . take a few moments to look this page over.
    PROBE: Would the information on this page be useful to you or anyone you know? (Who?) When would you want to have this kind of information in your hand?

        PROBE: Based on what you've read here, do you feel you know enough about what an HMO is? IF NO: What else would you want to know?
    PROBE: Based on what you've read here, do you feel you know enough about what MediPass is? IF NO: What else would you want to know?

Now let's look at page 3. (How do you use this booklet). (allow a few moments for participants to read the page)
    PROBE: Are these instructions clear? Do they give you a good idea of how this booklet can help you? IF NO: What should we change? (How?)

PROBE: Would you use a booklet like this if you had to chose a plan today?

PROBE: Who here use this booklet to choose a Medicaid plan, either for you or your child? How did you use it? What did you like about the booklet? What didn't you like. What else did you use when you chose a plan?

Let's turn to page 4 of the booklet. (Star page)
This page tells you what other people in the county thought overall of their health plan, and their overall rating of their regular doctor or nurse.

PROBE: What do the stars tell you?

PROBE: What do you think about the information on page 4. Do you think it is helpful to have this information when you need to choose a plan? (Why?)

PROBE: Do you trust this information? Do you think the stars tell you what you can expect if you choose that plan? How do the plans compare? What does that tell you?

Let's turn the page. (Page 5)

PROBE: Based on what you know right now, how do you think the county got the information in this booklet?

Page 5 lists the kinds of things other people have told us are important to them in choosing a health plan.

PROBE: Does this list include information you would want to know about a plan? (Why?) What's missing from this list? What's here that is not helpful to you?

PROBE: What do you think of the black boxes that are on the left side of each page? Do they help you to use this booklet? Are they confusing?

Turn to the next page, page 6 (MediPass) and look it over.

PROBE: What does this page tell you? What do the stars mean?

PROBE: Do you trust this information? (Why? Why not?)

PROBE: Do you think this page tells you what MediPass would be like for you? (Why? Why not?)

PROBE: Look at the box on the left. Would this box help you? Is it confusing?

PROBE: Look at the "tip" box at the bottom of the page. Did anyone read that box? Would this box help you?

PROBE: Is there any information on this page you think we should take off? (Why?)

Turn the page and let's look at the next plan (PCA).

PROBE: What does this page tell you? How did PCA rate?

PROBE: Does this look like a plan that would be good for you? (Why? Why not?)

PROBE: Look at the "tip" box at the bottom of the page. Did anyone read that box? Would this box help you?

PROBE: Is there any information we should add to this page (Why?)

Turn the page and let's look at the last plan (United HealthCare).

PROBE: What does this page tell you? How did United HealthCare rate?

PROBE: Does this look like a plan that would be good for you? (Why? Why not?)

PROBE: Look at the "tip" box at the bottom of the page. Did anyone read that box? Would this box help you?

PROBE: Is there any information we should add to this page (Why?)

PROBE: Does one of these plans look better to you than the others? (Which plan? Why?)

PROBE: Do you think it is good to have one plan on a page? Would you rather see all plans on a page?

PROBE: What do you think about the table? It's the same table for each plan. What should we change? (Why?) What is confusing to you (Why?). Do you think people you know would be helped by this information? (Why not?)

PROBE: Did this information help you chose a plan? How?

PROBE: What else do you want to know about the plans you can choose from?

Let's turn to page 9 (What else should you consider). (allow participants time to look page over)

PROBE: What should we take off this page? What should we add?

PROBE: Does the black box on the left help you? (Why not?)

PROBE: Do the questions on this page help you? Exactly how do they help you? Who used this to chose a plan? Do you think you would have picked a different plan without the booklet?

Let's turn to the last page (How was the survey done). (allow participants time to look page over)

PROBE: Do you care how the information in this booklet was collected?

PROBE: Can you trust the ratings of the plans? (Why? Why not?)

PROBE: What could we do to collect information you would trust?

PROBE: Do you think enough people gave information about each plan?

PROBE: Thinking about all the pages we just reviewed, how could we make this booklet better? (more useful to you)

PROBE: If you could add one more thing to the booklet, what would you add?

PROBE: Is there anything we should take out? (Why?)

IV. Alternate Formats for Presenting Survey Data (30 minutes)

A. HAND OUT MATRIX TABLE, GIVE PARTICIPANTS A MOMENT TO LOOK IT OVER

PROBE: What do you first notice when you look at this page? What do you read first?

PROBE: How many plans do you see on this page?

PROBE: Is this page easy to read? What do you think this page tells you?

PROBE: What do the stars mean to you? What does it mean to have one star? Two stars? (How do you know that? If we hadn't already talked about the stars is there enough information to what the stars mean?)

PROBE: Is this a helpful way for you to compare plans to each other?

B. HAND OUT DIMENSION TABLE, GIVE PARTICIPANTS A MOMENT TO LOOK IT OVER

PROBE: What do you first notice when you look at this page? What do you read first?

PROBE: How many plans do you see on this page?

PROBE: Is this page easy to read? What do you think this page tells you?

PROBE: What do the stars mean to you? What does it mean to have one star? Two stars? (How do you know that? If we hadn't already talked about the stars is there enough information to what the stars mean?)

Let's turn to the next page (page 4). . .
    PROBE: How is this page different?
Let's turn to the next page (page 6) . . .
    PROBE: How is this page different?
    PROBE: How many plans are on these 3 pages?
    PROBE: Is this a helpful way for you to compare plans to each other?

C. Look at this sheet (HOLD UP MATRIX) and compare it to this one (HOLD UP DIMENSION).
    PROBE: Which of these two is most helpful to you if you were choosing a plan?

IF ONE IS MORE HELPFUL, PROBE: Look at pages 6-8 in this booklet, and compare it to this (HOLD
    UP "MOST HELPFUL"). Which of these two is most helpful to you if you were choosing a plan?

V. Summing up (3 minutes)
    A. Final Thoughts/Questions
    B. Thanks
    C. Payment

Appendix D

**ALTERNATIVE DISPLAY FORMATS FOR PLAN COMPARISONS
TESTED IN FLORIDA MEDICAID FOCUS GROUPS**

Overall Rating of Health Plan

Plan Name	How the plans did
MediPass 1-800-940-4803 OR 1-904-238-4803	★★
PCA Family Health Plan 1-800-328-5804	★★
United HealthCare of Florida, Inc. 1-800-899-6550	★★

★★★ = This plan did better than other plans in your county.
★★ = This plan did average for plans in your county.
★ = This plan did less well than other plans in your county.

Dimension by Dimension Comparison 1

Overall Rating of Regular Doctor (or Nurse)

Plan Name	How the plans did
MediPass 1-800-940-4803 OR 1-904-238-4803	★★
PCA Family Health Plan 1-800-328-5804	★★
United HealthCare of Florida, Inc. 1-800-899-6550	★★

★★★ = This plan did better than other plans in your county.
★★ = This plan did average for plans in your county.
★ = This plan did less well than other plans in your county.

Dimension by Dimension Comparison 2

Choosing the Health Plan Again

Plan Name	How the plans did
MediPass 1-800-940-4803 OR 1-904-238-4803	★★★
PCA Family Health Plan 1-800-328-5804	★★
United HealthCare of Florida, Inc. 1-800-899-6550	★★

★★★ = This plan did better than other plans in your county.
★★ = This plan did average for plans in your county.
★ = This plan did less well than other plans in your county.

Getting the Care They Need

Plan Name	How the plans did
MediPass 1-800-940-4803 OR 1-904-238-4803	★★★
PCA Family Health Plan 1-800-328-5804	★★
United HealthCare of Florida, Inc. 1-800-899-6550	★

★★★ = This plan did better than other plans in your county.
★★ = This plan did average for plans in your county.
★ = This plan did less well than other plans in your county.

Dimension by Dimension Comparison 4

Getting Care Without Long Waits

Plan Name	How the plans did
MediPass 1-800-940-4803 OR 1-904-238-4803	★★★
PCA Family Health Plan 1-800-328-5804	★
United HealthCare of Florida, Inc. 1-800-899-6550	★★

★★★ = This plan did better than other plans in your county.
★★ = This plan did average for plans in your county.
★ = This plan did less well than other plans in your county.

Dimension by Dimension Comparison 5

Doctors (or Nurses) Communicating Well with Patients

Plan Name	How the plans did
MediPass 1-800-940-4803 OR 1-904-238-4803	★★
PCA Family Health Plan 1-800-328-5804	★★
United HealthCare of Florida, Inc. 1-800-899-6550	★

★★★ = This plan did better than other plans in your county.
★★ = This plan did average for plans in your county.
★ = This plan did less well than other plans in your county.

Dimension by Dimension Comparison 6

Doctors (or Nurses) Spending Enough Time with Patients and Knowing Their Medical History

Plan Name	How the plans did
MediPass 1-800-940-4803 OR 1-904-238-4803	★★
PCA Family Health Plan 1-800-328-5804	★★
United HealthCare of Florida, Inc. 1-800-899-6550	★

★★★ = This plan did better than other plans in your county.
★★ = This plan did average for plans in your county.
★ = This plan did less well than other plans in your county.

Doctors (or Nurses) Talking with Patients About Preventing Health Problems

Plan Name	How the plans did
MediPass 1-800-940-4803 OR 1-904-238-4803	★★
PCA Family Health Plan 1-800-328-5804	★★
United HealthCare of Florida, Inc. 1-800-899-6550	★★

★★★ = This plan did better than other plans in your county.
★★ = This plan did average for plans in your county.
★ = This plan did less well than other plans in your county.

Dimension by Dimension Comparison 8

Whether They Complained to Their Plan (more stars means fewer complaints)

Plan Name	How the plans did
MediPass 1-800-940-4803 OR 1-904-238-4803	★★★
PCA Family Health Plan 1-800-328-5804	★★
United HealthCare of Florida, Inc. 1-800-899-6550	★

★★★ = This plan did better than other plans in your county.
★★ = This plan did average for plans in your county.
★ = This plan did less well than other plans in your county.

Having Good Doctos (or Nurses) to Choose From

Plan Name	How the plans did
MediPass 1-800-940-4803 OR 1-904-238-4803	★★
PCA Family Health Plan 1-800-328-5804	★★
United HealthCare of Florida, Inc. 1-800-899-6550	★★

★★★ = This plan did better than other plans in your county.
★★ = This plan did average for plans in your county.
★ = This plan did less well than other plans in your county.

	MediPass 1-800-940-4803 OR 1-904-238-4803	PCA Family Health Plan 1-800-328-5804	United HealthCare of Florida, Inc. 1-800-899-6550

People were asked to give an overall rating for

	MediPass	PCA Family Health Plan	United HealthCare of Florida
Overall rating for their plan	★★	★★	★★
Overall ratings for their regular doctor (or nurse)	★★	★★	★★

How the plans did

People in this plan were also asked about

	MediPass	PCA Family Health Plan	United HealthCare of Florida
Choosing the health plan again	★★★	★★	★★
Getting the care they need	★★★	★★	★
Getting care without long waits	★★★	★	★★
Doctors (or nurses) communicating well with patients	★★	★★	★
Doctors (or nurses) spending enough time with patients and knowing their medical history	★★	★★	★
Doctors (or nurses) talking with patients about preventing health problems	★★	★★	★★
Whether they complained to their plan	★★★	★★	★
Having good doctors (or nurses) to choose from	★★	★★	★★

How the plans did

★★★ = This plan did better than other plans in your county.
★★ = This plan did average for plans in your county.
★ = This plan did less well than other plans in your county.

Matrix Comparison

Appendix E

**DATA COLLECTION FORM FOR OBSERVATIONS OF
DECISION HELPER USAGE IN DAYTONA BEACH**

FLORIDA OBSERVATION FORM

Form #: _____   Completed By: _____   Date: _____

OBS	Q1. ENTER START TIME OF SUBJECT'S DECISION HELPER USE:	Q2. DESCRIBE THE SITUATION UNDER WHICH SUBJECT USED THE DECISION HELPER: (CODE ALL THAT APPLY)	Q3. THIS RECORD SHOULD BE LINKED TO OBSERVATION NUMBERS:	Q4. WHO WAS THE PRIMARY USER OF THE DECISION HELPER?	Q5. OBSERVED GENDER:	Q6. OBSERVED ETHNICITY:	Q7. OBSERVED DURATION OF SUBJECT'S USE OF DECISION HELPER:	Q7. OBSERVED USE OF PRINTER:	Q8. ENTER END TIME OF SUBJECT'S DECISION HELPER USE:
1	ENTER TIME: _____ OR □ DON'T KNOW	□₁ R WAS ALONE *SKIP TO Q5* □₂ R WAS ACCOMPANIED BY ONE OR MORE CHILDREN WHO DID NOT PARTICIPATE IN THE USE OF THE DECISION HELPER. □₃ R WAS ACCOMPANIED BY ONE OR MORE CHILDREN WHO DID PARTICIPATE IN THE USE OF THE DECISION HELPER. □₄ R WAS ACCOMPANIED BY ONE OR MORE ADULTS WHO DID NOT PARTICIPATE IN THE USE OF THE DECISION HELPER. □₅ R WAS ACCOMPANIED BY ONE OR MORE ADULTS WHO DID PARTICIPATE IN THE USE OF THE DECISION HELPER.	ENTER # _____ ENTER # _____ ENTER # _____	□₁ THIS SUBJECT OR OBSERVATION # _____ OR □₂ ALL USED EQUALLY □₃ DON'T KNOW	□₁ FEMALE □₂ MALE □₃ NOT SURE	□₁ BLACK/AFRICAN AMERICAN □₂ HISPANIC/LATINO □₃ WHITE □₄ ASIAN □₅ OTHER □₆ NOT SURE	□₁ LESS THAN A MINUTE □₂ 1-5 MINUTES □₃ MORE THAN 5 MINUTES □₄ DON'T KNOW	□₁ YES, USED PRINTER □₂ NO, DID NOT USE PRINTER □₃ NOT SURE	ENTER TIME: _____ OR □ DON'T KNOW Q9. □ R HAD AT LEAST TWO SESSIONS OF USE
2	ENTER TIME: _____ OR □ DON'T KNOW	□₁ R WAS ALONE *SKIP TO Q5* □₂ R WAS ACCOMPANIED BY ONE OR MORE CHILDREN WHO DID NOT PARTICIPATE IN THE USE OF THE DECISION HELPER. □₃ R WAS ACCOMPANIED BY ONE OR MORE CHILDREN WHO DID PARTICIPATE IN THE USE OF THE DECISION HELPER. □₄ R WAS ACCOMPANIED BY ONE OR MORE ADULTS WHO DID NOT PARTICIPATE IN THE USE OF THE DECISION HELPER. □₅ R WAS ACCOMPANIED BY ONE OR MORE ADULTS WHO DID PARTICIPATE IN THE USE OF THE DECISION HELPER.	ENTER # _____ ENTER # _____ ENTER # _____	□₁ THIS SUBJECT OR OBSERVATION # _____ OR □₂ ALL USED EQUALLY □₃ DON'T KNOW	□₁ FEMALE □₂ MALE □₃ NOT SURE	□₁ BLACK/AFRICAN AMERICAN □₂ HISPANIC/LATINO □₃ WHITE □₄ ASIAN □₅ OTHER □₆ NOT SURE	□₁ LESS THAN A MINUTE □₂ 1-5 MINUTES □₃ MORE THAN 5 MINUTES □₄ DON'T KNOW	□₁ YES, USED PRINTER □₂ NO, DID NOT USE PRINTER □₃ NOT SURE	ENTER TIME: _____ OR □ DON'T KNOW Q9. □ R HAD AT LEAST TWO SESSIONS OF USE

Appendix F

EXIT INTERVIEW QUESTIONNAIRES FOR THE
DECISION HELPER FIELD TEST IN DAYTONA BEACH

ENTER START TIME:_____ **AM/PM**

Hi, my name is (INTERVIEWER NAME) and I work at RAND. I noticed you near the Decision Helper over there. I'd like to ask you a few questions about the helper do you have about 5 minutes? As a token of our thanks, everyone who completes the interview will receive $5.

SECTION A. ASK OF EVERYONE

*1.   What made you approach the Decision Helper? Did you:

CHECK ALL THAT APPLY

1 ☐   See it on an earlier visit this week,

2 ☐   Hear about it from your Public Assistance Specialist,

3 ☐   (See the poster in the lobby,)

4 ☐   Hear about it from a friend or family member,

5 ☐   See the computer,

6 ☐   Or something else? (PROBE FOR REASON)
ENTER VERBATIM:

_____

*2.   Have you already met with your Public Assistance Specialist today?

        ₁☐ YES, ALREADY MET WITH PUBLIC ASSISTANCE SPECIALIST

        ₂☐ NO, WAITING TO MEET WITH PUBLIC ASSISTANCE SPECIALIST

        ₃☐ R VOLUNTEERS: NO APPT. TODAY,
              JUST WAITING FOR A FRIEND/HERE TO PICK UP FORMS/ETC.

*3.   Is this the first time you've been to <u>this</u> center?

        ₁☐ YES → SKIP TO Q4

        ₂☐ NO

*3a.   How many times have you been to this center? (Your best guess is fine.)

        # TIMES: _____

*4.   Based on what you know right now, do you think the Decision Helper over there:

        ₁☐ Has information about all kinds of welfare benefits,

        ₂☐ Has information about Medicaid health plans,

        ₃☐ Or has some other information on it? (PROBE FOR WHAT)
        ENTER VERBATIM:

        _____

        ₄☐ R VOLUNTEERS: DON'T KNOW ENOUGH
              ABOUT DECISION HELPER TO ANSWER

*5.   Do you have Medicaid right now?

$_1$□ YES
$_2$□ NO → SKIP TO Q6

*5a.   Do you remember when you first got Medicaid? What month and year was that?
       INTERVIEWER: IF R DOESN'T KNOW MONTH, OK TO JUST ENTER YEAR.
       ENTER MONTH: _____   ENTER YEAR: 19_____

ALL WHO ANSWER Q.5a SKIP TO Q.7.

VERSION 1 QUESTIONS 6 THROUGH 11

*6.   Do you expect to qualify for Medicaid in Florida?

$_1$□ YES
$_2$□ NO

7.   Have you already picked a Medicaid health plan?

$_1$□ YES → SKIP TO Q12 ON NEXT PAGE
$_2$□ NO

8.   Do you need to pick a Medicaid health plan?

$_1$□ YES
$_2$□ NO → SKIP TO Q12 ON NEXT PAGE

9.   Have you started to think about how you would decide which Medicaid health
       plan to pick?

$_1$□ YES
$_2$□ NO

10. Have you ever gotten health care from any of these Medicaid health plans: MediPass, PCA Family Health Plan, or United HealthCare of Florida, Inc.?

₁☐ YES

₂☐ NO

₃☐ NOT SURE

11. Do you think you have enough information right now to pick a Medicaid health plan?

₁☐ YES

₂☐ NO

===

VERSION 2 QUESTIONS 6 THROUGH 11

6. Have you ever had Medicaid in Florida?

₁☐ YES

₂☐ NO

*7. Do you expect to qualify for Medicaid in Florida?

₁☐ YES

₂☐ NO

8. Have you ever had Medicaid in any other state?

₁☐ YES

₂☐ NO

9. Have you ever used a computer?

₁☐ YES

₂☐ NO

10. Have you ever used an ATM, an automated teller machine?

☐₁ YES
☐₂ NO

11. Have you ever played a video game?

☐₁ YES
☐₂ NO

══

*12. Did you use the Decision Helper at all today?

☐₁ YES → SKIP TO Q.15 ON NEXT PAGE
☐₂ NO

*13. Why not? (PROBE: What else?)

ENTER VERBATIM:

_____
_____
_____

*14. This next question is very important, and I will still pay you for the interview -- no matter what your answer is. Did you complete an interview like this a couple of weeks ago?

☐₁ YES
☐₂ NO

┌─────────────────┐
│ **THANK AND**   │
│ **PAY R**   │
└─────────────────┘

15.   Is today the first time you've used the Decision Helper?

   ₁☐ YES
   ₂☐ NO

16.   Did you think the Decision Helper was too long?

   ₁☐ YES
   ₂☐ NO
   ₃☐ NOT SURE/DIDN'T SPEND ENOUGH TIME TO SAY

17   How hard or easy was it for you to use the Decision Helper? Would you say:

   ₁☐ Very easy,
   ₂☐ Somewhat easy,
   ₃☐ Somewhat hard, or
   ₄☐ Very hard?

18.   What did you like <u>most</u> about the Decision Helper? PROBE: What else?

_____

19.   What did you like <u>least</u> about the Decision Helper? PROBE: What else?

_____

20.   Do you think the information on the Decision Helper would help you choose between the Medicaid health plans?

   ₁☐ YES → SKIP TO Q22
   ₂☐ NO

21.   Why not?

_____

22.   Do you remember seeing a screen that looked like this? SHOW R STARS
       SCREEN SAMPLE

       ₁☐ YES
       ₂☐ NO → SKIP TO Q25 ON NEXT PAGE

23.   Do you think that charts like this are:

       ₁☐ Very easy to understand,
       ₂☐ Somewhat easy understand,
       ₃☐ Somewhat hard to understand, or
       ₄☐ Very hard to understand?

24.   Would the information on this chart help you choose between the Medicaid
       health plans?

       ₁☐ YES
       ₂☐ NO

25. Did you print out any information from the Decision Helper to take home with you?

   ₁☐ YES
   ₂☐ NO
   ₃☐ R VOLUNTEERS: PRINTER BROKEN OR OUT OF PAPER

26. Do you think you'll come back and use the Decision Helper again?

   ₁☐ YES
   ₂☐ NO

27. This next question is very important, and I will still pay you for the interview -- no matter what your answer is Did you complete an interview like this a couple of weeks ago?

   ₁☐ YES
   ₂☐ NO

END OF INTERVIEW. THANK AND PAY R.

ENTER END TIME: _____ **AM/PM**

ENTER CASE ID

CAHPS EXIT INTERVIEW PAYMENT RECORD

FLORIDA FIELD OBSERVATION DATA COLLECTION

I certify that on I paid the respondent a payment of:

₁☐ $ _____ for a partial interview

OR

₂☐ $5 for a completed interview

Payment was made on ¡ ¡ / ¡ ¡ / ¡ ¡
              MONTH   DAY   YEAR

by   _____

            INTERVIEWER SIGNATURE

INTERVIEWER CHECK LIST:

$_1$☐ COMPLETE RESPONDENT PAYMENT
RECORD
$_2$☐ COMPLETE INTERVIEWER
OBSERVATIONS
$_3$☐ CODE CASE DISPOSITION

1. GENDER (BY OBSERVATION):

   $_1$☐ FEMALE

   $_2$☐ MALE

   $_3$☐ NOT SURE

2. ETHNICITY (BY OBSERVATION):

   $_1$☐ BLACK/AFRICAN AMERICAN

   $_2$☐ HISPANIC/LATINO

   $_3$☐ WHITE

   $_4$☐ ASIAN

   $_5$☐ OTHER

   $_6$☐ NOT SURE

3. DESCRIBE THE SITUATION UNDER WHICH R USED THE DECISION HELPER:

    (CHECK ALL THAT APPLY)

    $_1$ ☐ R WAS ALONE
    $_2$ ☐ R WAS ACCOMPANIED BY ONE OR MORE CHILDREN
    $_3$ ☐ R WAS ACCOMPANIED BY ONE OR MORE ADULTS
    $_4$ ☐ DON'T KNOW

4. DESCRIBE THE SITUATION UNDER WHICH YOU INTERVIEWED R:

    (CHECK ALL THAT APPLY)

    $_0$ ☐ NON-INTERVIEW CASE
    $_1$ ☐ R WAS ALONE
    $_2$ ☐ R WAS ACCOMPANIED BY ONE OR MORE CHILDREN
    $_3$ ☐ R WAS ACCOMPANIED BY ONE OR MORE ADULTS

5. HOW COOPERATIVE WAS R?

    $_0$ ☐ NON-INTERVIEW CASE
    $_1$ ☐ VERY
    $_2$ ☐ MODERATELY
    $_3$ ☐ SLIGHTLY
    $_4$ ☐ NOT AT ALL

6.   OVERALL, DO YOU THINK THE INFORMATION R GAVE YOU IS RELIABLE?

$_0$☐ NON-INTERVIEW CASE

$_1$☐ YES

$_2$☐ NO

7.   WERE ANY UNUSUAL OR SPECIAL CIRCUMSTANCES DURING THE
       INTERVIEW OR R'S USE OF THE DECISION HELPER? IF YES, DESCRIBE
       BRIEFLY.

_____

_____

_____

CASE SUMMARY SHEET

A. INTERVIEWER INITIALS:_____

B. DATE OF INTERVIEW:_____

C. CASE DISPOSITION:

    ₁ ☐ COMPLETE *(COMPLETE INTERVIEWER OBSERVATIONS)*

    ₂ ☐ PARTIAL *(COMPLETE INTERVIEWER OBSERVATIONS)*

    ₃ ☐ REFUSAL *(COMPLETE INTERVIEWER OBSERVATIONS)*

    ₄ ☐ INELIGIBLE - R IS A MINOR *(COMPLETE INTERVIEWER OBSERVATIONS)*

    ₅ ☐ LANGUAGE BARRIER (DID NOT SPEAK ENGLISH) *(COMPLETE INTERVIEWER OBSERVATIONS)*

    ₅ ☐ OTHER NON-INTERVIEW

D. IF CASE IS A REFUSAL, NOTE ANY REASON FOR REFUSAL (IF ONE GIVEN).

_____

_____

_____

DRAFT

Appendix G

INTERVIEW GUIDE FOR THE PROCESS EVALUATION
FLORIDA MEDICAID DEMONSTRATION

PROCESS EVALUATION SITE TOPIC GUIDE
Adapted for Use with the Florida Medicaid Program

December 16-18, 1997

HISTORY AND ORGANIZATION

History and experience providing consumer information for health plan choice.
History of the organization's involvement with health insurance and managed care plans.
Legislative and political context for Medicaid managed care.
Health plan enrollment process and use of choice counseling.
Experience conducting surveys in general.
Experience collecting data about beneficiary satisfaction.
Assistance from health plans with providing consumer information.
Intended audience for the information.
Actors/stakeholders in making decisions about benefits.
Other satisfaction or quality data available.
Scope of work for each vendor used.

PAPER REPORT INTERVENTIONS

Stakeholders involved or consulted in development and review of draft reports.
    Strengths:
    Weaknesses:

How results were presented to Medicaid recipients.
    Strengths:
    Weaknesses:

How information was marketed or disseminated.
    Strengths:
    Weaknesses:

Was intervention appropriate for the population.
    Strengths:
    Weaknesses:

What other information provided to Medicaid recipients.
    Strengths:
    Weaknesses:

How paper reports compare to any previous products.
    Strengths:
    Weaknesses:

Number of Medicaid recipients exposed to the information.
    Strengths:
    Weaknesses:

Who implemented the information interventions.
    Strengths:
    Weaknesses:

Type of publicity undertaken.
    Strengths:
    Weaknesses:

Design and implementation choices.
    Strengths:
    Weaknesses:

Why choices made.
    Strengths:
    Weaknesses:

Assistance site used or needed.
    Strengths:
    Weaknesses:

EVALUATION OF PAPER REPORTS

How was information intervention received by the target consumer populations?
Any other impacts as a result of the survey and information intervention?
Potential uses of CAHPS information in developing the choice counseling program?
Any other information or costs to pass on to other CAHPS users?

DECISION HELPER INTERVENTION

How well it operated on a daily basis.
    Strengths:
    Weaknesses:

Frequency of need to reboot, fill paper bin, call consultant, or other troubleshooting activity.
    Strengths:
    Weaknesses:

Effects on users of the economic services office.
    Strengths:
    Weaknesses:

Effects on staff serving the users of the economic services office.
    Strengths:
    Weaknesses:

Numbers and types of inquiries received about the decision helper.
    Strengths:
    Weaknesses:

Usefulness in informing new Medicaid recipients of health plans.
    Strengths:
    Weaknesses: